DEMENTIA
TOGETHER

How to Communicate
to Connect

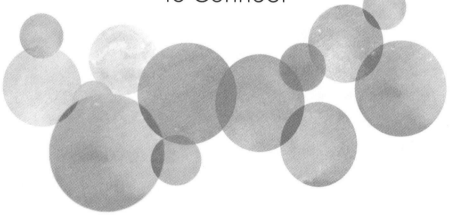

PATI BIELAK-SMITH

T0159359

PuddleDancer
PRESS

2240 Encinitas Blvd., Ste. D-911, Encinitas, CA 92024
email@PuddleDancer.com • www.PuddleDancer.com

Dementia Together: How to Communicate to Connect
© 2020 PuddleDancer Press
A PuddleDancer Press Book

PuddleDancer Press, Permissions Dept.
2240 Encinitas Blvd., Ste. D-911, Encinitas, CA 92024
Tel: 1-760-652-5754; Fax: 1-760-274-6400
www.NonviolentCommunication.com Email@PuddleDancer.com

Ordering Information
Please contact Independent Publishers Group, Tel: 312-337-0747; Fax: 312-337-5985;
Email: frontdesk@ipgbook.com, or visit www.IPGbook.com for other contact information
and details about ordering online.

Author: Pati Bielak-Smith
Foreword: © 2020 Bob Woods
Copyeditor: Tandem Editing LLC
Indexer: Beth Nauman-Montana
Cover and interior design: Lightbourne (BookWiseDesign.com)
Author photo: Yasoda Melville

Manufactured in the United States of America

1st Printing, January 2020

 Printed on recycled paper

24 23 22 21 20   2 3 4 5 6

ISBN: 978-1-934336-18-2

Library of Congress Cataloguing-in-Publication Data

Names: Bielak-Smith, Pati, author.
Title: Dementia together : how to communicate to connect / Pati Bielak-Smith.
Description: Encinitas, CA : PuddleDancer Press, 2020. | Series: Nonviolent communication
     guides
Identifiers: LCCN 2019019276| ISBN 9781934336182 (paperback) | ISBN 9781934336304
     (e-book pdf) | ISBN 9781934336366 (mobi/kindle)
Subjects: LCSH: Dementia--Patients--Care. | Dementia--Patients--Family relationships.
     | Alzheimer's disease--Patients--Care. | Alzheimer's disease--Patients--Family
     relationships. | Interpersonal communication. |
BISAC: HEALTH & FITNESS / Diseases / Alzheimer's & Dementia. | FAMILY &
     RELATIONSHIPS / Eldercare.
Classification: LCC RC521 .B538 2020 | DDC 616.8/31--dc23
LC record available at https://lccn.loc.gov/2019019276

ENDORSEMENTS OF *DEMENTIA TOGETHER*

"Emphasises how authentic relationships are at the heart of supporting someone with dementia. Makes a compelling case for how—with a curious and empathic approach to communicating—two-way connections can be enriched over time. Practical and humane, this book is recommended for anyone caring for or about a person with dementia."

—**TIM BEANLAND, PhD**, Head of Knowledge, Alzheimer's Society

"A vitally important and helpful book on an essential topic."

—**PETER J. CONRADI, PhD**, Fellow of the Royal Society of Literature and author of *Iris Murdoch: A Life*

"A book that acts as a guide in the richest sense: lucid, compassionate, and illuminating."

—**NICCI GERRARD**, award-winning journalist and author of *The Last Ocean: A Journey Through Memory and Forgetting*

"Many recent books have been written about dementia care but none attempt to understand the experience of dementia for the sufferer as well as *Dementia Together*. Pati Bielak-Smith's insights will be both practical and inspiring to professional and family caregivers who are often running to stand still in their caring roles and preoccupied with what the person with dementia cannot do rather than what they can."

—**DR. CLAIRE LAWTON**, consultant in old age psychiatry

"This delightful book introduces the reader to the possibility that dementia does not have to be the end of our relationship with a loved one but the beginning of a new and possibly an even closer one. For all of us, this book brings home how empathy is the key to a good relationship."

—**LAMA SHENPEN HOOKHAM, PhD**, author of *There Is More to Dying Than Death*

"This book changed my life in my relationship with my mother who has dementia. It has helped me find a heart-to-heart connection that allows me to communicate from a place of deep compassion. Through being curious about her experience, I can find meaning beneath what might otherwise make no sense. In connecting with curiosity and compassion, we can each feel heard and understood by the other. In some ways our relationship is closer than it has ever been."

—**RACHEL EDWARDS,** family caregiver

"A fascinating insight into dementia through the eyes of another health care assistant. A very interesting read, one that I highly recommend."

—SOPHIE ANN ELIZABETH McCLAY, professional caregiver

"This is a very sweet book about connecting with people who have dementia using empathy and honesty. All people who care for others need to read this book. Not only will it help you do a better job, but it will make your life more wonderful by decreasing stress and increasing enjoyment of the moment. By understanding how to listen to the meaning under the words and the behavior of people, you will save yourself a lot of angst judging people, creating separation, and adding more violence to the world, and you will be able to create intimacy and connection."

—MELANIE SEARS, RN, MBA, PhD, author of *Humanizing Health Care: Creating Cultures of Compassion With Nonviolent Communication*

"Written in a clear and confident style, with honesty, humility, and empathy based upon her own relationships with people living with dementia, the narrative is often poignant, sometimes funny, and always respectful, even when communication is tricky and connection seems elusive. The power of this book is in its honest simplicity and the heartfelt courage to share joint experiences and learning. We are invited to 'grow a bigger heart.' That's a challenge we can all aspire to, and at the end of the day, what we all hope we might be offered, especially if living with a dementia."

—DANUTA LIPIŃSKA, National Dementia Care Award winner, and author of *Dementia, Sex and Wellbeing*

"*Contented Dementia* by Oliver James opened my eyes to new ways of thinking about dementia care. This book by Pati Bielak-Smith goes much further, with real practical approaches that will help carers, families, and professionals develop better ways to work with people who have this condition."

—DR. AVRIL DANCZAK, FRCGP FRCP AoME BSc PGCE, GP/primary care medical educator and lead author of *Mapping Uncertainty in Medicine: What Do You Do When You Don't Know What to Do?*

DEDICATION

To my Granny Irena
For daring to be vulnerable

To Mahatma Ghandi
For daring to be nonviolent

CONTENTS

Foreword by Professor Bob Woods · ix

Introduction: Growing Connection · 1

PART ONE: SEEING RELATIONSHIP

1 Acknowledging What's There · 11

2 Focusing Imagination · 27

3 Getting Perspective · 45

4 Committing to Life · 69

PART TWO: TASTING FOR YOURSELF

5 Cultivating Empathy · 87

6 Feeding Inner Power · 109

7 Savoring Hurt, Guilt, and Grief · 121

PART THREE: LISTENING WITH HEART

8 Being Curious · 139

9 Tuning In to Anger and Confusion · 157

10 Asking Questions · 171

11 Staying in Touch · 185

Endnote: Experiencing Vulnerability   193

Epilogue: Expressing Gratitude Without a Tail   197

Acknowledgments   201

Appendix A: Resources for Dementia and
        Nonviolent Communication   205

Appendix B: Dementia-Friendly Empathy   207

References and Recommended Reading   209

Index   217

The Four-Part Nonviolent Communication Process   221

About Nonviolent Communication   222

About PuddleDancer Press   223

About the Center for Nonviolent Communication   224

Trade Books From PuddleDancer Press   225

Trade Booklets From PuddleDancer Press   232

About the Author   234

FOREWORD

Dementia is arguably one of the great challenges faced by humanity in the first half of the twenty-first century, alongside the likes of climate change, civil wars, and population migration. Alzheimer's Disease International estimates that the current figure of 46.8 million people around the world living with dementia will increase to 131.5 million by the year 2050. These figures include those who have one or more of the various disorders (including Alzheimer's disease and vascular dementia) that lead to changes in day-to-day life related to impairment in memory and other mental abilities and are characterized as dementia. An equivalent number of family members and friends will take on caregiving roles, which are known to increase the risk of mental and physical health difficulties.

There are glimmers of hope in these figures. The increase in the number of people affected is due to more people around the world living longer, into the age groups (seventy-five years and older) where the risk of developing a dementia is greatest. Yet there are signs that the proportion of people affected by dementia at any given age may be falling. This may be due to better heart health as well as better education. Reductions in smoking and improvements in exercise and dietary habits, as well as social and mental stimulation, form part of a raft of potentially preventative actions that could lead to estimates of the number of people affected by dementia being revised downward in the future. And although the current available medications have limited effects, there is a massive global effort to find disease-modifying treatments, which may eventually also make a difference.

Whatever the future holds, however, many millions of people will live to experience a dementia, and here the hope is to find ways in which people with dementia may experience well-being and quality of life, despite the changes being experienced. There are already tangible indications that this hope can be realized. Over the last decade, people diagnosed with dementia have become prominent self-advocates, speaking to the media, writing best-selling books, and contributing in a meaningful way to policy and service development. There are not just a few exceptional individuals; there are networks of self-help and peer support groups in the United States, Canada, the United Kingdom, and across Europe, all with the same message: There is life after a dementia diagnosis. Alongside the social movement to create dementia-friendly communities, these networks have begun to change the way we view people with dementia. As a result, we are witnessing the beginnings of a massive change in public attitudes and awareness.

People with dementia tell us that they do not always "live well with dementia." They are not immune from anxiety, low mood, frustration, anger, distress, uncertainty, self-doubt, despair, insecurity, fears for the future, or grief for what has been and is being lost. As memory becomes more impaired and communication becomes more difficult, managing the range of emotions that are a normal part of the human experience becomes more challenging.

Having to depend on others can be difficult, and this loss of independence can be experienced as a threat to the person's identity and autonomy. The social psychologist Tom Kitwood has described how to maintain the "personhood" of the person with dementia, in the face of dementia-related changes, by providing care and support in a way that values the person as an individual, offers a positive social environment, and seeks to understand the world from the perspective of that person. This approach, usually described as *person-centered care*, has been a dominant influence in the development of higher-quality care and support for people with dementia around the world.

Sadly, however, it appears that many people with dementia do not receive or experience person-centered care. Although simple in concept, person-centered care can be very difficult to implement in practice, and this book gets to the heart of why this is the case and what you can do about it.

As Kitwood pointed out, person-centered care relies on the relationship between the person with dementia and the person in the caregiving role. There are then (at least) two parties involved, and the personality, sensitivity, empathy, understanding, fears, anxieties, insecurities, and losses of the caregiver are just as important to the outcome of caregiving as is the cognitive impairment of the person with dementia.

Some experts in dementia care have thus preferred the term *relationship-centered care* to *person-centered care*, and some have tried to make a distinction between the two. In my view, Kitwood's idea of person-centered care was always founded on relationships; he saw personhood as being upheld (or conversely diminished) in the context of relationships, with cognitive impairment making it necessary for others to help maintain the person's identity and memories and to validate their feelings.

In this book, Pati Bielak-Smith shares with us powerful, moving stories from her experience as a live-in caregiver and the intense relationships she formed with people living with dementia. These stories illustrate the need to understand and acknowledge the pathway through life and experiences that have shaped the person we see now. Pati's emphasis on communication and on connection helps each of us to face the challenges of making person-centered (or relationship-centered) care a reality. Communication is not just about "getting through" to the person with dementia, and it is certainly not about "making them understand." It is a two-way process, involving the caregiver in attentive listening: listening to the words, listening to the silences, listening to the nonverbal communication, and above all listening sensitively to the emotions underlying what is being communicated.

It was some years ago now that Naomi Feil, in her writing and teaching on validation therapy, first advocated listening to the feelings of people with dementia. She also stressed the need for the caregiver to be centered and put aside other distractions so that full, undivided attention could be given to the challenge of communication, interaction, and connection at a deep human level—described by Kitwood as "I-thou" relating. These messages remain timely and important and in this book are found embedded in a framework many will find helpful.

This framework that underpins Pati's work, Nonviolent Communication, is one that I had not encountered previously in the field of dementia care. Generally, I am averse to concepts that are defined by what they are not. For example, I prefer to talk about psychosocial interventions rather than nonpharmacological interventions. At first sight of the term *nonviolent communication*, a caregiver may be tempted to say they are already doing this: after all, they are never "violent" to the person in their care.

Yes, sometimes they are rushed and don't have time to explain, sometimes they realize their words sound patronizing, sometimes it takes physical effort to get the person changed into dry clothes if they are resistant, sometimes medication has to be given to quiet the person down . . . but violent, never.

However, it is worth going beyond the label to discover that in the framework laid out in this book, communication is seen as an exchange that brings *connection*. Many of the principles and techniques are very appropriate to the context of dementia care, including the discovery of playfulness in relationships, where humor and joy can at times be found in the simplest of interactions. But ultimately it seems Nonviolent Communication is about peace. Helping people living and dying with dementia—and those who support them—to find peace of mind is an aim that is incredibly worthwhile, and we should use every means available to endeavor to achieve it.

BOB WOODS

Emeritus Professor of Clinical Psychology of Older People,
Dementia Services Development Centre Wales,
Bangor University, United Kingdom

Growing Connection

Dementia surprised me.

Before I had any real experience with it, I thought of it as something "old"—concerning the elderly—and something to do with dying. I also thought it affected a "small" number of people and was insignificant in the grand scale of things.

Then I learned I was mistaken, on both counts. Working with people who have dementia turned my perception of it upside down—I learned that dementia is the opposite of what I had originally thought.

Three letters describe my early experience with dementia: NEW. It wasn't negative, it wasn't positive, it was simply something previously unknown to me. Poignant. Despite people talking about dementia as "a slow death" and "a deadly disease," my experience of people with this illness instead enriched my life. I also believe that my relationship with them brought more life into their experience.

I am not the only one who has encountered this surprising spark of life. One relative of a person with dementia told me she found a new window of communication with her mother due to the illness. Their experience with dementia together was both scary-new, but also fresh-new. The kind of freshness that comes with feeling alive. Even after having some experience of being and working with different people who have dementia, I still find this freshness. The experience does not wear off, but it remains new, as you never know quite what to expect—including who will be affected, when, and precisely how. Among other things, there are more and more cases of dementia being diagnosed among people in their thirties and forties. (So, my perception of dementia as "old" was also incorrect.)

My second surprise was in learning the significance of dementia to the world. Again, three letters are enough to describe the scale: BIG. It's big not only in terms of the number of people affected, and the expectations for the number of people who will be affected in the future, but also in terms of the enormous impact dementia has on the personal lives of the people diagnosed and those who are close to them.

About fifty million people worldwide have Alzheimer's or other types of dementia. This book is for the fifty million people who love, care about, or care for the first fifty million. Because every person with dementia, at some stage of their illness, will have at least one person who cares for them. And usually, more than one person who cares about them. That means there are certainly no fewer than one hundred million people affected by dementia right now, directly or indirectly.

When I talk about caregivers in this book, I mean not only those who deliver care or care *for* someone, but also those who simply care *about* someone who has dementia.

I am one of the people who cared for somebody with dementia. For five years, I cared for several people with dementia. I am not a health care specialist, nor a nurse or doctor, nor a scholar. But as a professional caregiver of people with dementia, I experienced many of the day-to-day challenges of life with dementia: behind closed doors (when politeness to visitors has worn off), after medical professionals have left (when people stop being on their best behavior), and at strange times of day (when one can no longer distinguish day from night).

Throughout this book, I share some of the ways that dementia has affected my life, both professionally as a caregiver and personally as a great-granddaughter. I found that whether dementia is experienced in a professional capacity or in family life, it is always a very personal matter. The approach of those who care for someone with the illness should therefore also be personal. Each relationship is different, but at the same time each is a helping relationship in which help is being offered and received, in a manner that is skillful or not. This help exchange places communication skills at the very heart of the relationship.

Carl Rogers, one of the founders of the humanistic approach to psychology, devoted a large proportion of his research to formulating the components of a helping relationship. His research showed that helping is fundamentally associated with a relationship between two people: "A helping relationship might be defined as one in which one of the participants intends that there should come about, in one or both parties, more appreciation of . . . the latent inner resources of the individual."

Caregiving in its very essence is a helping relationship. Sadly we often think of caregiving simply as a service provided to someone who is suffering. As a one-way street. This is an assumption that I challenge in this book.

Dementia indeed challenges many of our usual ways of seeing the world. Back when I faced my first challenge, in my great-grandmother's vascular dementia, I thought dementia was related to death. After all, dementia is what took my Grandma Maria away. More recently, I have learned that there is more to dementia than loss. In fact, my relationships with my clients who had dementia enriched my life, brought more aliveness into my work, and made my heart grow. What I discovered is that because dementia is so BIG, to measure up to the challenge, my heart had to grow bigger.

When I began working as a professional caregiver, I had already started learning Nonviolent Communication. Nonviolent Communication taught me to see communication as not a one-way but a two-way street. By honoring this fact, I learned that I could connect with another person far more easily. And that everyone gains from this connection.

Marshall B. Rosenberg, who founded the Center for Nonviolent Communication in 1984, created Nonviolent Communication as a process that rests on key ideas of the helping relationship described by Carl Rogers. Rosenberg added depth by drawing on principles from wisdom traditions around the world, such as Judaism, Christianity, Sufism, and Buddhism: "All that has been integrated into Nonviolent Communication has been known for centuries about consciousness, language, communication skills, and use of power that enable us to maintain a perspective of empathy for ourselves and others, even under trying conditions."

I think it is fair to say that life with dementia provides plenty of trying conditions. When I began working with my first dementia client, I desperately needed some context to help me understand what was happening. It was a matter of necessity that I put these two things together—what I learned during my eight years of Nonviolent Communication training, and what I learned during the five years I provided professional care to people with dementia.

During that time, I had many opportunities to learn how to use Nonviolent Communication in daily life with people who have dementia. At times I found it lifesaving.

I wrote this book to help caregivers, friends, or family members of someone who has dementia to find more ease, life, and connection in their relationships. The perspectives and principles presented in this book have been echoed by other Nonviolent Communication teachers and practitioners around the globe who are related to someone with dementia or who work with them in a professional capacity.

Stories in the book come from England and Wales (where my work is based) and from other countries, as I interviewed Nonviolent Communication practitioners living in the United States, Australia, and throughout continental Europe who had also found this approach invaluable. By using Nonviolent Communication skills, we have restored relationships we thought were permanently damaged by dementia and created new relationships with people who were said to be unable to assimilate new information. Throughout this experience, we learned from each other—from our allies in Nonviolent Communication practice and from those who have dementia. Because it's a two-way street.

The characters you will meet in this book are real people, though the names of those with dementia, as well as some personal details, have been changed to protect their anonymity. Every effort has been made to provide the essence of these interactions with people who have dementia, without giving away too much of their private information. Hence all stories are told primarily in my own words, whether they are based on remembered conversations or recorded interviews. Some of the Nonviolent Communication practitioners I interviewed opted to remain anonymous, and others allowed me to use their real names.

We have found that there *is* a way to reach a satisfying and deeply connecting relationship between two people, even when dementia is a condition affecting one of them. It does not deny difficult emotions or daily challenges, but uses them to build solid ground for connection. We may not be able to affect the course of someone's illness, but we can cultivate a healthy relationship that enriches both our lives throughout our time together. This is what I call *dementia relationship:* a relationship that has more to do with life and growth than with diminishing capacities or cognitive deficits. In this relationship both people's needs—those of the caregiver and the cared for—are being taken into consideration and matter equally.

In this book, you will read stories about communication that creates connection between two people. The kind of connection that encompasses both giving compassionately and receiving empathically, because in Nonviolent Communication, both sides matter.

If these stories inspire you, you may be interested in pursuing further training in Nonviolent Communication. This is a skill that can be strengthened progressively over time through regular practice. See Appendix A for information about learning opportunities offered by Nonviolent Communication teachers around the world, both in person and online.

Even if you decide not to pursue further training in Nonviolent Communication, reading the chapters in this book will help you learn principles that will redirect your experience with dementia— to focus more on life than on the illness. The primary principle on which this book rests is that communication is about connection.

The first part of the book, Seeing Relationship, explains why connection is so important in a relationship with someone who has dementia.

The second part, Tasting for Yourself, explores ways to connect with yourself, value your own needs, and delight in self-empathy.

The last part, Listening With Heart, is devoted to ways to connect with someone who has dementia.

Dementia challenges our habitual ways of seeing things. Life with dementia can be distressing and scary, and much of the time really frustrating. But you don't have to lose your senses. Focusing your communication on connecting with the person who has dementia can bring you both back to life. You will see beyond what seems obvious. You will wake up and smell the roses, taste the sweetness of connection, listen with heart, and pronounce your presence through touch. Because, as a poet once remarked, "the universe is full of magical things patiently waiting for our senses to awaken."

PART ONE

SEEING RELATIONSHIP

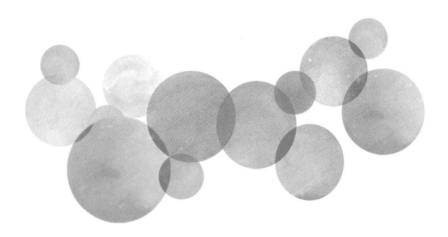

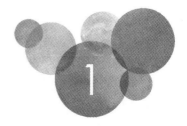

Acknowledging What's There

But what am I going to see? I don't know.
In a certain sense, it depends on you.

—STANISŁAW LEM, *Polish writer*

Lucia is a friend of mine who emigrated from South America at a young age. Now living and working in Europe, she sees her mother only once a year. On one visit, she arrived to find that her mother was showing signs of dementia.

"Where are you? Are you there?"

"Yes, Mum, I'm right here."

"I can't see you."

"That's because your eyes are closed. To see me you need to open your eyes."

Lucia's mother forgot that she has to lift her eyelids to be able to see. Due to dementia she has lost this basic knowledge.

Dementia is a word that describes a group of symptoms that result from damage to the brain caused by disease. Dementia can be caused by several different factors affecting the brain. The symptoms are progressive, usually beginning slowly and imperceptibly, with the effects getting more pronounced over time, sometimes gradually and sometimes rapidly depending on the cause.

Many people experience the illness as losing a loved one bit by bit, with the loved one withdrawing as the people who care about them give up. We associate dementia with parting ways, moving away, leaving for good.

You wouldn't abandon your loved one, but you may feel as if your loved one has left you already. You may feel lonely when you lose a connection that you once shared, or a connection you always hoped for. It may feel like it's too late. This is one way of seeing the situation—but it's like seeing it with your eyes closed. Or filled with tears.

Eyes are windows to your soul. A pained soul keeps the blinds down. But if you don't open your eyes, you won't let the light in. You won't notice that the person you care about is still there, and so is your relationship with them. But the first step is to acknowledge their dementia.

WHAT OFTEN GOES UNSEEN

We often do not see four essential elements:

First, dementia itself. It is an invisible sort of illness; it does not reveal itself through bandages, wheelchairs, or walking aids. It starts slowly. It is subtle. It is a different experience for each person it affects. We don't necessarily know if someone has dementia by looking at them. That's how invisible dementia is.

Second, the person behind dementia. Because once dementia is diagnosed, it is all too easy to pay more attention to the disease than to the person who has it.

Third, the caregiver behind the person behind dementia.

Fourth, the relationship between those two people. There is still, always, a relationship between a person with dementia and a person who cares for them.

Dementia itself is difficult to spot in the wild. It affects people subtly, even in its advanced stages. But eventually, things start disappearing. Almost imperceptibly, particular skills, words, and knowledge may start to vanish. Even so, which skills a person loses, and to what extent, differs from person to person. This means there is no "standard" form of dementia. However, loss of memory and loss of words are two ways that people commonly recognize dementia.

An average adult knows about thirty thousand words. What difference does it make if someone forgets a couple of hundred of them? It is not immediately obvious—neither to the person who has dementia nor to the people around them. Work by famous authors such as Agatha Christie, Iris Murdoch, and Terry Pratchett showed symptoms of language deterioration before the authors themselves were aware of the disease. Not even their most faithful fans noticed, at the time. The study of these writers' novels did not take place until after they were diagnosed with dementia, or in some cases even after their deaths.

Time is another subtle clue. Saint Augustine famously stated, "What then is time? If no one asks me, I know what it is. If I wish to explain it to him who asks, I do not know." No wonder people with dementia get confused about time—time of year, time of day, or time of their life. They aren't quite sure what year it is. They get day and night mixed up. And like most of us, they feel younger on the inside than they appear on the outside. Unlike the rest of us, they may believe that if they feel twenty, they must *be* twenty.

A person who seems to be losing things more and more often—words, keys, and sometimes their temper—will at some point be taken to the doctor. As they enter, they are treated like a regular person, though perhaps as a person who's a little forgetful. They are addressed directly, in first person: Take a seat, Mr. Jones. But after they have been diagnosed, they are discussed in third person, as if they are not there: We are afraid that Mr. Jones is showing signs of Alzheimer's. Once dementia has been acknowledged, it takes over the show. The diagnosis often marks the transition between not seeing dementia to seeing *only* dementia.

Why have you started talking about me as if I weren't in the room? Mr. Jones might ask. This is the moment when a person seems to disappear behind dementia. Like one person I used to know.

A PERSON HIDDEN BEHIND DEMENTIA

Dementia can act like a cap of invisibility: whoever has it turns invisible. Indeed, someone who has had dementia for a while can mysteriously go unnoticed in the midst of their family's everyday life. A person with dementia is unable to contribute much in terms of housework, is incapable of following conversations in the usual way, and is often deprived of their personal friendships, leading them to retreat into the background. In my family, that person was my great-grandmother, known in my family as Grandma Maria.

I was in my teens when I realized I knew hardly anything about Grandma Maria, who was at the time in her nineties. She lived with her daughter, my Granny Irena, in an old two-bedroom flat which I visited on a weekly basis, and yet I could not recall seeing Grandma Maria much. She was always quiet, like a shadow. She was used to keeping out of the way, I suppose. I only spotted her moving silently between her bedroom and the neighboring bathroom, and once a year around the Christmas table, where she sat without saying a word.

Everyone in the family seemed to treat Grandma Maria with respect, but silently, from a distance, and without talking to her. I don't recall many interactions I had with her, apart from one meaningful conversation. Later in the book, we will explore the odd mechanics of human memory, one of them being that we tend to remember things that have personal significance for us. The event I'm about to share with you wasn't a particularly big one in the sense that no one can validate it for me; it wasn't a significant part of my family history. But it was meaningful for me, as it illustrates how I lost my great-grandmother even before she died. In a sense, she passed away from my world years before she actually died, and in my personal history, this was an event worth remembering.

At some point in my teens, I began to realize how little I knew about this mysterious ancestor of mine, and I became determined to spend some time in her company. My sudden interest might have been ignited by a family tree project at school. I remember the amazed responses from my friends whenever I mentioned that I had a living great-grandmother who was nearly a hundred. At that time it was very unusual to have such an ancient relative. And mind you, we were only one generation away from those who had lived through the Second World War. In fact, my great-grandmother had lived through two world wars—a dubious privilege.

I decided there was no time to be wasted. Although I already paid regular visits to Granny Irena's house, there was only one occasion when I remember going specifically to see Grandma Maria.

That day I knocked and went into her room, asking politely whether I could join her for a moment. I had a secret mission to claim my heritage. To me, as a teenager, she was the living past. She looked like the past. She behaved, sounded, and even smelled like the past. Walking through the door into her room was almost like time travel, like being teleported into a living, breathing history, more alive than any old history book, yet smelling the same. This was it, my chance to have a real conversation with my own great-grandmother!

I will never forget her bright face and sheer delight at welcoming me into her room, her kingdom. She seemed attentive and observant, yet there was something passive about her. She didn't say anything as I came in, nor did she offer me a seat. I sat down next to her on the sofa bed.

I started by asking a series of questions about her life and our family. She became engaged, smiling and sitting up a little bit. She told me about some cousins of hers in Poland who had fled to a remote part of the country, in the North, after the Second World War, and how much she wished she had visited them there.

Curious, I asked her more questions. I asked what games children played during her time. I asked whether there was any television back then, and what would she do in the evenings without it? In response she said: "After the war, my cousins fled to the North. All my life I wished I had gone to visit them."

I froze in confusion. Didn't she realize she was repeating herself? I thought maybe she hadn't heard me. Old people tend to go deaf, I thought. So I asked her about the television again, and she retold the whole story about her cousins all over again, as if it were the first time.

I lost interest almost immediately. I was so confused, and embarrassed because I didn't know how to react. The worst thing was that I felt utterly disconnected from her. I felt separate and detached, almost as if we were strangers rather than family. It was an uncomfortable sort of feeling, like when you feel utterly alone despite being with someone.

Grandma Maria and I were in the same room physically, but I felt very distant from her.

She seemed stuck in the past, and although I was interested in her personal history, I couldn't understand why she went around in circles about the same topic. I was interested in comparing the past to the present, but she didn't seem to know anything about the present.

We were so far apart that our sentences could not travel through time to make communication possible. What was the point of talking then?

If she doesn't realize what she's saying, she probably doesn't understand who I am, or where we are, or what any of this means, I thought. I not only withdrew my interest but I also lost any feeling of warmth or closeness. I kept nodding, while looking for any opportunity to leave the room. In a very strange way, I felt as if she had rejected me, simply because she repeated the same story several times.

This repetition, and worse, the fact that she was oblivious to it, made me question everything about our relationship. And the point of it. Tragically, I began to see her as a robot—a machine lacking awareness or any meaning whatsoever, mechanically repeating the same old story. She was simply parroting a story that was etched in her mind as a series of information bytes inherited from the person she used to be, or so I thought. At the time, I felt that her lack of short-term memory meant that she too was gone.

I left the room as politely as I had entered it, but this time I crossed the threshold without hope.

Afterward, I simply glossed over the whole experience with one convenient judgment: Oh, well. She's just old. Little did I know at the time, my great-grandmother was living with dementia, most likely vascular dementia that developed after her stroke. I don't know whether knowledge of a medical condition would have influenced my experience in her room back then. I suspect I would have glossed over it with only a slightly different understanding: Oh, well. She's got dementia. Meaning, there's nothing I can do about it, so I will continue to politely acknowledge her existence without any hope for connection.

She may have lost her mind, but I was the one who lost heart. And that is how we lost one another.

It doesn't have to be that way.

This book exists to share what I've learned and practiced about how to maintain heart, connection, and communication with someone one who has dementia. To do it, you need to see the person behind dementia and see another person too: yourself.

A CAREGIVER OUT OF SIGHT

Dementia caregivers can be just as invisible to people around them as those with dementia are invisible, because it is not immediately obvious that someone with dementia requires care.

Unlike a small child who cannot be separated from their caregiver. If we see a small child alone in a public place, we wonder where their parent is. Where is their mother, father, or any caregiver for that matter? We expect them to be visible. Children need caregivers for food and shelter, to keep them safe. Just as fundamentally, children need adults for companionship—to hear their needs, and to laugh, play, and fight with them. Every child needs someone to communicate with, and to connect with. When we see a child alone, we assume something is missing—or rather someone.

Caregivers to those with dementia are so invisible to the public that people wouldn't even notice if they are missing. And yet they are no less essential. People with dementia are not children. Yet behind every person with dementia, there is a caregiver. If we see someone who has advance dementia unaccompanied in a public place, would we ask ourselves: Where is their caregiver?

We probably wouldn't. Unless we had some experience of how dementia can disable someone's abilities, we wouldn't be alarmed to see them alone, would we? Not in the same way as if we saw a child on their own.

And yet, the caregiver of a person with dementia is an essential component of their life—just as a parent is an essential component of childhood. Except that caregivers of people with dementia have the added difficulty of being invisible to the world, and even the person they care for. Their job is not obvious to people who don't realize what dementia care requires.

Caregivers are life-enablers. And yet most of the time this caregiving role is as invisible as the disease itself. Do we wonder how someone with dementia gets through the day, every day? Do we wonder who prepared their food when they forgot how to open the refrigerator, or when they forgot they needed to eat food in the first place? Who answers one question after another, often the same question all day long?

People don't demonstrate dementia in any obvious way, and therefore they do not appear disabled. Not even, or maybe especially not, to their own eyes. I'm fine, Mr. Jones might say—I do all these things on my own. Having forgotten that bills have to be paid, and pets need feeding, they may not comprehend why they wouldn't be able to cope by themselves. And indeed, in early stages of the disease, many people who have dementia can manage well on their own and won't need a caregiver for daily personal care or to keep them safe. But this won't last.

Sooner or later, people with dementia lose the ability to do daily tasks like cooking a meal, doing laundry, driving, or handling money. They may not be aware of it because along with the skill goes their sense of necessity for daily tasks. But their caregiver will be aware. Their caregiver will notice and be able to help in more than one way.

Caregiving can mean hands-on work helping another with everything that everyday life involves. It can also, just as importantly, mean organizing and masterminding direct care providers while managing everything else in a person's modern life, from paying bills to answering emails. When I talk about caregivers in this book, I mean not only those who deliver care but also those who simply care about someone who has dementia—in this book I use "care for" to mean both types of caregiving. Either of these forms of care involve a to-do list that is longer than the hours in the day.

Did I ever notice the caregiver of Grandma Maria? Did I ever wonder who listened to her repetitive story about her family's venture to the North? Who made sure she had everything she needed from morning till night? Did I ever realize Granny Irena was her sole caregiver? I knew Granny Irena well, and I loved her with all my heart, but I did not recognize the caregiving she devoted so much time to. It was invisible, in the background. The caregiving involved smooth and continuous hours of care—around the clock.

So on top of the endless tasks that care itself involves, a caregiver has to deal with being invisible—to the world at large, to passersby, and even friends and family who do not notice dementia happening at all. Invisible even to the very person they are caring for, since people are often unaware of their own dementia, and therefore also unaware of the role of the person who was "just" their husband or wife, son or daughter, friend or neighbor. They may not realize that now they are caregivers too.

Caregiving can happen so invisibly that a caregiver may even be invisible to themselves. They may not realize they have taken on this additional role, with its additional cost. When a caregiver ignores their own needs and the things that matter to them personally—perhaps unaware of how they could possibly meet everyone's needs in the situation—they end up burned out and downhearted. And, perhaps most painfully, they become disconnected from the very people they do all of this work for.

Care describes something that happens between two people, yet for many people, caregiving feels solitary. Expectations are high on all sides. People expect a caregiver to be compassionate, resourceful, and have an endless supply of patience—under any circumstances, always. Is that what you expect of yourself?

The job of caregiving is, as the word implies, all about giving. Giving time, effort, and attention. It may seem like you're giving much more than you're receiving, and that your lonely one-way street gets only steeper and more winding over time.

What I hope you learn while reading this book is to open your eyes not only to what you need yourself, but to how much you are, or could be, *receiving*. In other words, to learn not only how to be more efficient at giving love and care, but also how to receive something precious from the people you care for. How to enrich *your* life.

RELATIONSHIP AS A TWO-WAY STREET

This book, and all of my work with people who have dementia, is based on the discipline of Nonviolent Communication. Nonviolent Communication teaches people to connect with each other by learning not only how to give compassionately, but also how to receive gracefully. In communication, this translates into honestly expressing and empathically receiving.

If you already offer care, love, or respect to another person, do you also know how to receive it from them? In a relationship with a person who has dementia, there may be many blocks in communication, like barriers in language or perception, but that doesn't mean they have nothing to offer you.

Communication is at the heart of every relationship, and in its very essence, communication is a two-way street. If I have one hope for this book, it is to help you learn how to get more out of your relationship with someone who has dementia.

People with dementia, though they require care, are not children. They can be partners in caregiving, helping you help them and supporting you in many ways. People with dementia so often long to contribute in a meaningful way. Anthony de Mello, a Jesuit priest, said that old people are often lonely not because they have no one to share their burden, but because they have only their own burden to share. To me this explains why so many people with dementia feel useless and alone: because they wish they could contribute meaningfully.

Even when someone can't realistically *do* much to contribute in the household, they can still *be* in relationship with you. Meaningful contribution can be delivered with their heart, not only with their hands.

I wish I had been able to see my own great-grandmother behind her dementia. I wish we'd been able to have the type of relationship I've had since then with other people who have dementia. Instead I was told that "she's out of her mind" and "she's not all there." So where was she then? I didn't know where to look for her, how to meet her where she was. I was lost. And because of that, I lost Grandma Maria. My inability to communicate caused the untimely death of our connection. She became even more absent from my life after our memorable conversation than before, as if she had died to me, even though she lived on in her body for another two years.

Dementia didn't kill our connection, however. It was my own disconnection that had such deadly consequences for our relationship. Once we acknowledge the disconnection that sets us apart from other people, we can do something about it.

DISHEARTENING DISCONNECTION

Dementia can affect thinking and memory in a range of ways. It can affect day-to-day, recent memory. It can cause difficulties with planning, concentrating, or organizing. It can affect use of language. It can affect visuospatial skills. It can affect orientation to time or place. Sometimes it causes visual hallucinations or delusions. Dementia can also lead to changes in mood, but *dementia does not cause disconnection.*

Disconnection is a state of having a closed heart and a disengaged mind.

The various symptoms of dementia, such as emotional withdrawal, volatility, or decreased attention and motivation, are often associated with disconnection. But disconnection is not an inevitable part of dementia.

Disconnection means disengagement that can lead to loosening of bonds with people. In contrast to the sense of life that a meaningful connection with another person can bring about, disconnection cuts off these bonds. It robs people of the aliveness that comes with connectedness in life, and they eventually drift away from others. Although they may be spending a lot of time physically close to other people, they are not necessarily present in their spirit. For those who feel disconnected there isn't much "closeness" about the quality of that time.

It is disheartening when disconnection happens. Disconnection can occur equally on the part of the person who has dementia as well as anyone around them. It can take place in any relationship and between any two people, with or without dementia. It is disconnection, not dementia itself, that leads to the sense of isolation, loneliness, and separation that many people living with dementia experience. In many cases disconnection is the most painful factor in living with dementia. And this pain can lead to making dementia even worse than it has to be. The worse off someone is in their heart and spirit, the more dependent they become, and the more care they require, and the less cooperation there will be. Eventually, disconnection costs everyone more time, effort, money, and heartache. Who pays these costs? In most cases the caregiver pays the price for disconnection, making their work and their relationship even more painful. It isn't in anyone's interest to ignore disconnection.

Acknowledging disconnection when it occurs can reveal options that would stay closed otherwise. Like a question that never gets answered unless someone asks it.

Asking how you can connect with the person who has dementia can spark imagination. I am not asking you to imagine impossible things—on the contrary, I invite you to dream of the possible, the actual and genuine. Dream with your eyes wide open and feet firmly on the ground. There is a way into a satisfying and deeply connecting relationship between two people, even when one of them has dementia. In the next chapter I will share four stories from my life about such connections. The rest of this book will explain how you can communicate to connect with the person you care for.

Lucia and her mother managed to save their relationship despite the challenges of dementia, geographical distance, and the different lifestyles and cultures they ended up living in. Lucia knew that her ability to save their relationship was not a matter of being lucky. She used the discipline of Nonviolent Communication and her spiritual practice to see through the illness and maintain a quality of connection with her mother. It was a matter of skills and a bigger perspective. A little bit of imagination helped too.

Dementia can deprive one of many skills, abilities, and memories, but it does not have to deprive us of connection. "It is true what they say, you know—that connection never dies," Lucia said to me. "In a sense, I have never really lost my mother."

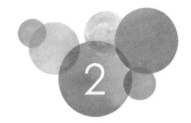

Focusing Imagination

You can't depend on your eyes when
your imagination is out of focus.

—MARK TWAIN, *American author*

What's the first step to making something happen? The very first step is to picture it as a possibility. In this way you set your eyes on the destination: a satisfying relationship with someone who has dementia. A relationship which keeps your connection alive.

Such a relationship requires both imagination and compassion. With imagination, we consider how others might experience the world. With compassion, we focus on how their experience of the world affects them. If imagination is the mind's eye, then compassion is the heart's eye. In a relationship with someone who has dementia, we need both.

Indeed, when dealing with dementia, we often need to draw on all resources available.

IMAGINATIVE COMMUNICATION

Starting with a pinch of imagination can be very helpful when trying to decipher some of the unusual behaviors associated with dementia. In fact, imagination might be one of our mind's best tools for reaching out to others, for understanding what appears to be beyond understanding.

You cannot assume that a person affected by dementia perceives the world the same way you do. You might see a bath filled with bubbles. They might see a boiling volcano. Imagine that. When it's hard to get your head around what's happening, focus your imagination. For clues about how dementia is affecting the person in front of you, pay attention to how they relate to the world around them.

Both of you will be affected by what you perceive in different ways. That warm bath full of bubbles may appear very comfy to you, but very scary to someone with dementia who fears losing control and wants to guard their intimacy and autonomy. Besides, who would want to get into a volcano naked? That would be rather uncomfortable.

Yet the very same person may be perfectly comfortable wearing their underwear not underneath all their other clothes, but on top, whereas you would find such a situation embarrassing and might long for a bit of consideration.

Dare to imagine how another person might be feeling, what they might be needing, and how you might be able to contribute to their well-being. Without forgetting yourself either. You're growing a heart big enough to understand both perspectives, and a mind resourceful enough to find solutions that would work for both you and the person you care for.

In this chapter, I will tell you some stories that come from my relationships with four people who have dementia. Each one of them required full-time care, due to their dementia and often to other accompanying conditions. I stayed with them in their homes, as a professional caregiver, for several weeks at a time. As I shared their lives for that time, in a sense I shared a life with dementia. And I learned how it can affect everyone involved.

We need our hearts to understand both perspectives, and our minds to find solutions that work for everyone.

Each person I cared for was affected by the disease in a different way. I have learned that there is no "standard" or "by the book" case of dementia. Dementia occurs in people over age sixty-five, and in younger people too. It can disable someone from recalling what happened only five minutes ago, while they have no problem describing in detail something that happened fifty years ago. One person with dementia may be unable to hear what you say to them right in their ear, while another may be disturbed by the distant noise of a plane eight thousand feet above them. Dementia is full of paradoxes. Nobody who has it seems to feel obliged to follow any "rules" of the disease—as if there were any in the first place! Instead, each person might as well be saying: I will do this illness my way, thank you very much.

One very important characteristic of dementia is that its symptoms are likely to be inconsistent even in one person alone. Some of my clients had severe memory or perception problems one moment, only to be entirely clear-minded the very next moment. For a caregiver, this is both unsettling and lifesaving. It is unsettling because it keeps you on your toes: you can never know quite what ability or disability to expect. Yet this inconsistency also gives you many second chances to approach a scenario more skillfully. If things didn't go well the first time you tried, you can try, try again.

Using your imagination on a daily basis could make your care routine more exciting, leaving room for some unpredictability.

It is unimaginative to assume that because someone can't make a decision one day, they will never be able to make that decision, or that they have lost the ability altogether. Yet too often, tragically, people try to treat someone with dementia "equally," where "equal treatment" means treating someone in each case as if it were their worst day. Approaching someone with dementia from this perspective can be both debilitating and deeply depressing. This chapter explores how to approach someone with imaginative openness instead.

So now I have the pleasure of introducing you to my unpredictable clients: Gordon, Clare, Dory, and Yvonne. Four people with dementia with whom I formed dementia relationships. I spent more time with some than others, and some relationships felt more personal than others, but in each case my client and I figured out how to relate to each other in a way that created a meaningful connection. Sometimes quite unexpectedly.

Ultimately, these four people were my best trainers in imaginative communication skills. They taught me how dementia can affect people's ability to remember, view, observe, and foresee reality, as well as how it indirectly affects caregivers—in this case, how their dementia affected me.

THE MAN WHO FOCUSED MY IMAGINATION

Gordon had worked for half a century as a village vet, and along with his wife, Jenny, he shared a dislike of the city lifestyle. They had both been very hands-on country people, managing their land

and their household together until Gordon's health deteriorated after a stroke that resulted in early onset of Alzheimer's and reduced mobility. Since that time, Gordon needed company whenever Jenny could not be with him.

He walked slowly, and I had to walk with him and watch his steps, as he had fallen several times in the past. Also, when walking, he often stopped abruptly and watched the floor very attentively.

The first time I noted this, we were on our way to his bedroom, both rather tired at the end of the day. He stopped for no apparent reason, and I tried to be patient and encouraging. "Gordon, we're nearly there," I said. "We just need to cross the hall."

He did not respond, but maintained his attentive gaze on the mosaic of the corridor floor. I wondered whether he had suddenly felt some pain, or maybe he had stopped to remember something, because I couldn't see anything on the floor he might be staring at.

In other words, I couldn't see what he was seeing.

So I reminded myself: When my eyes are of no use, let me try my imagination. And instead of hurrying him up, I paid attention. I became interested. I focused my eyes right where he was looking.

Paying close attention to someone is like paying a visit to their world.

Perhaps this focused attention encouraged Gordon to explore further, because he then moved his right leg forward, tapping the area under analysis with his foot, as if double-checking the surface. Then he suddenly remarked, "You know, for whatever reason, my brain wants me to believe there is a hole in front of me. Right here, you see? But I can feel with my foot that it is a solid surface. How very odd!"

Gordon found the way that his senses presented the world to him to be very amusing, and he began to share these observations with me. Each time was a discovery for him and an amazement to me that he had this double perspective. On one hand, he saw black holes all around him, but on the other hand, he was able to question whether they were truly there. He was relaxed, not disturbed by it. Just a little bemused each time.

What I learned from this experience is that a person's observation is less important than their response to it. Gordon was amused. Everyone needs fun in their life, and Gordon's study of the holes in his floor met this need for him.

When he shared this amusement with me, he also met a need for companionship. I wouldn't, on my own, have conceived that a perfectly even floor could be taken for a bottomless black hole. But I could imagine that this was surprising and even in some way fascinating. I could also imagine that to someone who did not have Gordon's curiosity and confidence, such faithlessness on the part of the floor might be frightening—something worth bearing in mind the next time you witness someone hesitating to cross a black doormat or a patterned carpet. Their stuckness may not be a matter of stubbornness but an inner battle between reason and perception. Is the abyss real? Should I fear it, or have the nerve to walk across it? The answer depends not only on what they see but also on how they see it. Frightening or entertaining? There is only a fine line between the two.

I admit that some days I was not excited at the prospect of examining the floor again. There were always household chores, more or less urgent, that needed doing. And sometimes I was simply worn out. I often chatted with Gordon over supper, and at times I expressed what was on my mind or how I was feeling. After I shared what bothered me, Gordon rarely needed any extra prompting from me. I did not need to hurry him up. If he was aware that I had no extra time that day, he slalomed around the black holes in the floor without discussing the status of their existence. He did not need to be reassured, calmed down, or convinced that the holes weren't there. It was easier to walk around them.

To connect with Gordon, I had to meet him in his world. I had to visit him there, through the power of my imagination. My mind's eye then allowed my heart's eye to hear his feelings of amusement and wonder. I was imagining, he was seeing, and through this connection, both of us were able to enjoy a sense of companionship.

With Gordon I learned that connection is possible even between people who are not necessarily the best of friends. We two had our differences, in worldviews and life philosophies. His favorite hobby had been shooting animals for sport, whereas I was horrified by the idea of killing a sentient being. But we had a good time together. A friendly relationship is not the same as a friendship, and yet both can connect two people in peaceful companionship.

THE WOMAN WHO MISTOOK ME FOR A PHONE

Clare's natural environment was her garden. It was her creation, and something that kept her alive in return. After many years of a demanding career in banking, she changed gears and chose to retire in a secluded area. She thrived on being surrounded by greenery and beautifully kept grounds, which made it even more unfortunate that her vascular dementia affected her vision. She was still able to encompass the view over her carefully designed flower beds and rows of bushes, but smaller details had become more difficult to comprehend.

She lived alone, and I stayed with her for several different periods over the course of a year, witnessing all four seasons of her garden. I learned that Clare's ability to see individual objects clearly, and to recognize them for what they were, was more changeable than the weather.

One day as we sat in the living room doing crosswords, Clare dozed off as usual. I continued doing crosswords in my book on the table, with Clare drowsing next to me in her armchair. Suddenly she woke up and looked around. She looked at me but right through me—she didn't seem to see me at all, even though I was only an arm's length away from her.

She grabbed my left hand from the table and lifted it.

I froze, not knowing what was going on. But I didn't make any sudden moves, not wanting to scare her. Judging from the look on her face, she wasn't aware I was even in the room.

She put my hand next to her ear and said, "Hello?"

Once I realized that she had mistaken my hand for a telephone, I said, as gently as I could, "Clare, I am here."

She continued talking to the phone. "What? Where are you? Speak louder!" In her own quiet manner, she was, in fact, shouting at my hand.

"I am right here," I said, and I moved toward the center of her field of vision. (I later learned her vision was better on her left side, while I had been sitting on her right side that day.)

When Clare saw my face, and that there was a hand attached to it, she was not amused. She hid her face in her own hands in resignation and gave a deep sigh. She may have felt stupid, or indignant. Instead of laughing it away, or trying to convince her that nothing had happened, I tried to imagine what it might have felt like for Clare and empathized the best I could. "You seem dismayed . . . Is that because you would like to understand what just happened?"

While Clare may have lost some of her visual skills, she never lost sight of her own needs. On many occasions, I heard her mourn her loss of vision and long for clarity and understanding. We went to medical doctors and optometrists, and she explained to them and to me that "the objects around me keep moving; they don't stay the same." A phone suddenly becomes a person, for example. Many other times she mistook me for a hairbrush or a chair to sit on. My arms were mistaken for a belt to put around her waist. To me this proved a point made by Gerald Edelman, an American biologist, who said that every act of perception is to some degree an act of creation, because it depends so much on both what we see and also how we interpret what we see. In his book *The Man Who Mistook His Wife for a Hat*, Oliver Sacks describes neurological cases of patients who misinterpreted people for objects, and vice versa, similar to how Clare confused my hand for something else entirely.

Clare was worried and perplexed, as anyone might be in such circumstances. After several conversations, together, we guessed that her worry arose from her need for safety and dignity. Understanding her unmet need was important. I had to do more than imagine her feelings of confusion, perplexity, and fear. It was when we recognized that she longed to feel safe in the world—"which moves around a lot"—that we were able to come up with ideas to make this world safer and more stable for her.

One strategy was for me to say, "Hi, Clare. I'm here, by the window"—or wherever I was at the time—as soon as she entered a room where I was. Before I was mistaken for a phone, I hadn't imagined that I would not be visible to someone who wasn't blind. I had assumed she would see me for herself.

I also moved my armchair to sit on her left, where she could see me more clearly. And whenever I addressed her, I held her hand. This provided her with a sense of support, an arm she could lean on, something stable and reliable.

These strategies helped, but the primary building block contributing to Clare's sense of safety was our communication, and the trust that we built over time. Communication and trust made it possible for us to come up with doable solutions that we could introduce straightaway. They were specific, as in, "When I talk to you, I will hold your hand so that you know where I am, and that I am next to you." These little things created a bond between us, on many levels. And they helped me realize that Clare was good at growing many kinds of things, including our professional relationship, which grew into friendship.

This relationship met my need for contribution and mutuality so deeply that often I felt more uplifted and replenished after spending time at Clare's than when I had my time off. Many times we switched roles in a sense. If I confided in her that I was suffering from period pain or was in a low mood, she expressed genuine empathy and care. She cared about me, though of course she did not care *for* me. If Clare offered me a cup of tea for comfort, I was the one who made the tea. Did that matter? I had more physical ability and more trustworthy eyesight, but care went both ways between us. We cared about each other.

When two people connect through communication and trust, both people are more likely to be flexible, imaginative with solutions, and willing to stretch a little. But sometimes you hit a boundary, a situation you are not willing to go along with. This is a time to say no.

THE WOMAN WHO HEARD MUSIC IN MY NO

Dory was a retired music teacher whose passion for music led her to live a short distance from a concert hall. As close as it was, it wasn't within walking distance, and public transport wasn't conveniently available. She needed a car to get there.

Although Dory was the fittest of all my clients, both physically and mentally, she was also the least aware of her dementia.

Her mental abilities, such as understanding her surroundings, multitasking, problem-solving, and decision-making, were seriously compromised, and Dory herself was almost utterly unaware of her brain condition. She was very well aware of her other health problems, such as sensitive skin and heart arrhythmia, but she appeared to know nothing about her Alzheimer's. She would even forget she had forgotten about it.

But her family and friends (of whom she had many) were aware of her condition. They also recalled the story of a man with dementia who drove into a group of people crossing the street, because he confused the accelerator for the brake.

When Dory's trusted friends got together with her to discuss her declining ability to drive, she eventually made the sensible decision to sell her car. At the time, with everyone present and with all facts on the table, Dory, I was told, had been perfectly okay with making this decision, which was documented in writing with her signature on it.

After a very short time, all these facts had left Dory's head for good. The absence of her car was highly upsetting, and any attempt to present her with the written documentation of the circumstances and reasons for selling the car unnerved her. Family and friends made all the necessary arrangements for Dory to be able to attend her weekly concerts, and this was regularly erased from her memory.

When I met Dory, she was still very tormented about the car, which she noticed missing on a daily basis. "You see now that I don't have a car, I can't go to concerts anymore," she would say. "I haven't listened to live music for months now. Would you help me get my car back?"

Her observation wasn't factually accurate: she had not missed any concerts since the car was sold. The loss of her own vehicle was not preventing her from going to the events. Furthermore, getting the car back was practically impossible and something I wasn't willing to help her do anyway. I shared her family's concern for her safety and the safety of others around her.

So far, the situation seemed impossible to solve because it was based on a false assumption and an inaccurate observation, and it involved a demand I didn't want to fulfill.

Assumption: "Now that I don't have a car, I can't go to the concerts." (Not accurate.)

Observation: "I haven't listened to live music for months now." (Not accurate.)

Demand: "Help me get my car back." (I said no.)

I was unable to make Dory see the inaccurate assumptions and observations she was making without confronting her, or questioning her sanity. I felt frustrated that there was no reasonable way to explain to Dory why she could not drive again. How I wished for some understanding on her part! I was stuck, and annoyed— until I realized that instead of trying to convince Dory about how mistaken she was, I could simply listen to what mattered to her the most.

What I learned from Dory was that to be on the same page with her, I needed to address directly the very thing she cared about the most. Safety wasn't Dory's primary interest. What mattered to Dory was that she could trust there would be a way to get to her concerts.

In other words, I didn't need to get stuck in my own false assumption that the only way forward was for Dory to understand *my* reasons and observations. Instead, her ability to reason could be replaced with her ability to connect.

Listening to Dory made me realize that live music was so important because it was, in a sense, keeping her alive. Without

music, there was no point to her life; that's
how meaningful music was to her. The car
was simply the strategy that she associated
with the thing she lived for—music.

*The ability
to reason can
be replaced with
the ability to
connect.*

This made sense to me. I was able to
understand what was beneath her anxiety
about the car and her longing to attend
musical events.

The first conversation with Dory in which I expressed genuine
interest in the importance of music seemed to settle her a lot. She
felt heard and understood. But she then made the assumption that
because I understood, I was therefore going to get her car back. It is
so easy to jump to the conclusion that someone who understands us
will do what we want.

But Dory's need for feeling alive and uplifted wasn't the whole
picture. I also had my own needs, such as for ease and safety. And I
was going to say no to Dory's wish for her old car.

I once watched a television program about hotel services, and
how staff members were trained to never say no to a client. One
receptionist said it was his personal ambition to never refuse his
client anything, whatever they wanted. I thought to myself: What
is so frightening, or offensive, about saying no? I suppose people
may think that saying no can imply a lack of respect, or lack of
consideration to someone's needs. The lesson I learned was that if
I am not prepared to go along with someone's request or demand,
ensuring the person knows I care about their needs will help
our relationship. If I acknowledge my own needs too, we become
partners in our relationship.

So I said no to Dory. I said no, I would not help her get her car
back. I stressed that I cared about Dory's needs as well as mine.
That I wanted to support her in getting to the musical concerts, and

that I would be so much more relaxed if we drove in my car. Saying no to helping her get the old car back was my way of saying yes to a relaxed time together, when we could both enjoy the beauty of live music. "How does that sound?" I asked her.

Upon hearing this, Dory seemed touched. "Would you really enjoy taking me? It would be wonderful to share the time together, and it would free me of the trouble of getting my old car back," she said. Hearing the pleasure I took in supporting her to stay connected to her musical passions was in itself music to her ears. In truth, she didn't care about the car at all. Once we were able to get to the bottom of this—her passion and my need for safety—we found a solution in no time.

This solution was not a new one. In a sense, we reinvented the wheel because it wasn't the first time Dory had been driven to a concert by her caregiver. But this time, she was easy about it. And she stopped mentioning her car so often afterward. Connecting to both of our needs kept us on the same page even when facts and assumptions were unreliable and fleeting. Our connection was, in a sense, unforgettable.

Dory didn't remember my name, nor did she know who I was or what I was doing in her house. She didn't think I was her caregiver, because to her best knowledge, she didn't require any care. However, because of the connection we made with each other, she assumed I was a friend. In her mind, why else would she feel warm toward me, and why would I be staying at her house? People tend to be kind to their friends, cooperative and easygoing, and open to discussion and different solutions. They care what their friends need. She wasn't thinking of herself as a customer at a posh hotel where every wish was a command. Rather, we were friends. At home. Together.

In this way, I and other friends involved in caring for Dory met her needs while also fulfilling our own values of contribution, collaboration, and friendship.

THE WOMAN WHO PUT MY IMAGINATION TO THE TEST

"You're being thrown in the deep end with this client," I was told when assigned to work as a caregiver to Yvonne. "Your soft approach won't work with this one. You have to make sure you follow the procedures to cover your ass in case there's a complaint. This client has made complaints against caregivers in the past, so watch yourself."

Yvonne was once an owner of a highly rated beauty salon, but since living with dementia she was better known for her "challenging behavior." This judgment was based on the numerous occasions when she had expressed her agitation by hitting, or at least trying to hit, the people around her. During her latest stay at the hospital, Yvonne had been aggressive toward staff members and had often been tamed with drugs. Now back at home, still bedridden, she was getting her strength back. But she had not yet recovered from her fury.

That night, as I was about to take over from the previous caregiver, I heard her screaming, "Take me home at once! Can you hear me?! Get me out of here! You wretched, stupid woman!"

Yvonne was in a state of anguish, which she was expressing through violence and verbal abuse toward the caregiver who was desperately trying to calm her down in her bedroom. I made my way in to investigate, and I witnessed a conversation in which any attempt to make a clear observation failed tragically.

"But you *are* in your own bedroom. Look around," said the caregiver in a loving voice, trying not to contradict the woman who could not recognize the bedroom in which she had slept for the last thirty years. "Look at the picture of your late husband. You recognize him, don't you?"

"You stupid woman! This is *not* my bedroom!"

At this point Yvonne's tantrum reached its peak as she tried her best to be aggressive, even while her weak, ninety-seven-year-old hands failed to succeed at what she intended: to hit her caregiver. She was ready to persuade the caregiver by force that her own perception of the room was correct.

Whatever Yvonne was observing was not being acknowledged. But even if the caregiver played along with Yvonne's delusion, how could she do what Yvonne was demanding? How could she take Yvonne "home" when they were home already?

I exchanged looks with the caregiver. I could see she was at the end of her wits; she'd had a long day. And Yvonne's demand was simply impossible to satisfy. But let's try it anyway, I thought.

After pausing for a few minutes, I approached Yvonne, who was helplessly waiting to be saved from the bed in which she had spent countless nights over the last few decades. Pausing usually helps to cool the heat of the moment, helps the storyline to fade a little. But the anger was still there, smoldering.

"Are you upset, Yvonne, because you feel you are not being heard?" I asked.

"I just want to be taken home. At once."

"I would like to help you do this—but I need your help, as I don't know how to get you home. I don't know where it is."

"That's all right, I know how to get there," she said. "Will you take me?"

The tone of her voice changed immediately. She had gone from seeing me as a caregiver—since she was unable to differentiate faces, we represented a function—to seeing me as an ally. Simply engaging with her about what made sense to her, without confronting her with facts, made her relax. She felt understood, and so already there was a certain level of connection. That's how our cooperation began.

"Let's get you in the wheelchair so that you can show me how to find your home," I said.

Now she was acting as if we were setting off on an adventure, sailing off into unknown waters, with me turning the wheel and her setting the direction. Her power and sense of self-governance was back with her. She was at home with feeling in charge.

We headed through the corridor and out the front door. Looking back at the house from the garden outside, she said to me, "That's my house, you see!" As if all this time she had been kept elsewhere, in some other, unfriendly place where she was powerless and useless. Now, feeling empowered and useful, she also felt at home. It was right there. As the novelist Cecelia Ahern has said, home isn't really a place, it's a feeling.

Yvonne wanted to show me around her newly discovered family home, where I was treated more like a guest. We went back through the same front door we'd left several minutes earlier, except this time Yvonne guided me through the corridor—she knew the place well—and back to the bedroom, which not long ago had felt like an unfamiliar place. But now it felt like home.

She became thankful, warm, and calm, treating me like a friend. Although in many ways I still remained a function to her, at least I was a useful, friendly function. A function she treated more like a human than a robot performing tasks.

Yvonne went to sleep within minutes of me putting her to bed. I was relieved and astonished and, admittedly, I giggled to myself. What a way to meet a need for autonomy! I would have never imagined!

Since then, Yvonne astonished me many more times. Gradually, she began to recognize me as a person, and became very attentive to my needs. "Go and rest your legs, dear. You must be tired," she would say after we came back from a stroll in her wheelchair through the neighborhood. She frequently offered me gifts, which I later put back in her jewelry box, so that she could offer them again soon after, without any recollection that we had done this exchange before. I never kept any of these objects; instead, I confess, I kept something far more precious—our connection.

I kept that connection close, right through the outbursts of anger or fear we experienced again and again, the periods of constipation and diarrhea, the bed falls and hallucination highs, the expressions of love and hate. It was rarely easy. And yet, from a bigger perspective, it was so worth it.

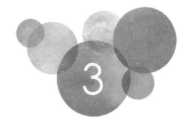

Getting Perspective

And maybe the big picture [is] amazing,
but if you're standing with your face pressed up
against a bunch of black dots, it's really hard to tell.

—REBECCA STEAD, *American author*

L iving with dementia is hard, for everyone involved. Yet it is possible to have healthy relationships, even when living with this illness. It's possible to have what I call a dementia relationship that is full of life, despite the dementia. And healthy relationships create well-being for both people in the relationship. However, many people who have been directly or indirectly affected by dementia find that an ill state of being is far more common than well-functioning relationships. There is a person with dementia, and a person close to them—two disconnected and mistrustful parties in the same relationship, trying to deal with, manage, and troubleshoot the real challenges of life with dementia. Close, yet so painfully apart.

This book is about seeing the possibility of reconnection. It offers new perspectives on living with dementia. It does not promise easy solutions, but instead simple solutions that make life more wholesome and far more meaningful.

There is a way to look at things which makes things simpler, without simplifying the problems. Seeing new possibilities is not only a matter of *what* we see and don't see, but also *how* we see—the perspective we have. When we gain greater perspective, it is easier to see how things are connected, and hence how we can connect with each other.

In everyday life, it's common for dementia caregivers to get lost in endless to-do tasks, demands, and newly emerging problems. In the midst of all this, it's easy to lose perspective on what really matters. Everyone gets confused: the person with dementia may not possess the mental faculty to comprehend clearly, and the caregiver may be under so much pressure, they find it hard to think, or even feel, clearly. And when we are confused, we forget about the bigger picture.

A BIGGER PICTURE

Marshall B. Rosenberg, the founder of Nonviolent Communication, liked to use the giraffe as a symbol of the bigger perspective that Nonviolent Communication brings. The giraffe is gentle but strong. It possesses the biggest heart among all land animals, making it a suitable image for a discipline that can help you grow your heart bigger, both in strength and in gentleness. And of course, we all associate giraffes with their long, long necks—which enables them to reach higher, to the very tops of the trees, and see farther than their short-necked companions on the savanna. Giraffes have a more all-encompassing view.

Similarly, by practicing Nonviolent Communication, we can access a bigger picture of every situation. We can even, in a sense, see into the future—because it is easier to foresee the outcomes of our interactions with others. We can imagine what will happen when we are skillful in communication, and what is likely to take place when we are not skillful. Like someone who sees dark clouds heading their way and says, "Close the windows. The storm is coming," we can become not fortune-tellers, but damage-preventers.

To prevent damage in any relationship, it is good to have a look around and see how we can make it stronger. This is why it is worth seeking ways to connect with one another—because being together strengthens each person.

Dementia affects both people in a relationship, even if only one has the illness. And each person affects the other. Examining what causes disconnection will give us a better sense of what leads to connection. Learning how to connect will put us in a better position to get more out of our relationships, including those with someone who has dementia. Connection makes compassionate giving effortless and makes empathic receiving inevitable. To get there, it's important to acknowledge that both parties contribute—to the relationship, and to the difficulties of living with dementia.

THE DEMENTIA RELATIONSHIP

Dementia caregivers often talk about the illness as a problem which belongs to *them*. It is they who need to be dealt with, looked after, managed, or protected. This way of looking at the situation makes an assumption that *they*—those with dementia—are the source of the problem.

Consequently, *we*—those without dementia who "know better"—have a problem with *them*. As Tom Kitwood and Kathleen Bredin wrote:

Here there is a clear division between *us* (members of the "normal" population), and *them* (the dementia sufferers). *We* are basically sound, undamaged, competent, kind. *They* are in a bad way, for they are afflicted. . . . So there is a need for training to give us knowledge about *their* illness, and to develop skills, especially in managing *their* "challenging behaviours."

Kitwood and Bredin then point out another way of looking at the situation with dementia, which is to consider this question: Whose problem is it?

Or, in my situation, if someone with dementia decides to pee into the sink instead of the toilet, who has more of a problem with it, him or me?

Gordon was affected by dementia in a way that made it difficult for him to orient himself spatially. On one hand, he saw holes in the ground that weren't there. On the other hand, he was frequently unable to locate objects that were actually there: Where was the door handle? How does one find a light switch? Where could one find a toilet to pee into?

Since all of these objects were hiding from his perception, he had found ways to do without them. The door to the bathroom attached to his bedroom was left permanently open, the light switched on at all times, day and night, whether he needed it or not. And as the toilet was never to be found, he developed a habit of using the sink to urinate into. The sink was much easier to locate, as it stood at a height that allowed him to feel it without needing to bend. The sink was so much easier!

So he peed in the sink, and with the stopper in place, the urine stayed there overnight, permeating the air of his bedroom such that I was attacked by a piercing smell every morning as I entered his room. As if Gordon himself was attacking me with his secret weapon. And the secret to this weapon was that it was neither sharp nor shooting, it neither hurt my skin nor fired bullets. Instead, it was disgusting. I sighed silently to myself. Why are you doing this to me, Gordon?

This unhygienic and smelly habit did not bother Gordon, a man keen on wearing clean clothes every day—a spotless, freshly ironed shirt and perfectly matching cardigan and trousers. He was clean and neat, *and* he didn't mind urine in the sink.

I did, though. I had a problem with it. I would be so embarrassed if someone walked into my bathroom and saw my bladder fluid. But Gordon wasn't embarrassed. It didn't affect him. And I assumed he didn't care whether it affected me or not—hence I judged him as inconsiderate and filthy. Sometimes I even thought to myself that he had "lost it altogether." These judgments only contributed to the problem. In a sense, I made the situation worse for both of us.

I thought I had to continue living with Gordon's disgusting habit, and perhaps more painfully, with my judgmental and disconnecting thoughts. Then one day I found out from his other caregiver that it was she who requested that he urinate in the sink!

She had known him longer than I had, and apparently, because Gordon was unable to locate the toilet in the middle of the night, he had frequently urinated all over the bathroom floor. So his caregiver requested that he at least aim for the sink, and thus save her a lot of work in the morning. I never considered that he was trying to collaborate, but instead I interpreted it as a nuisance. I assumed that he was being uncooperative, whereas all this time he was trying his very best.

After adjusting to this new perspective, the only thing that still bothered me about using the sink as a toilet bowl was that the stopper was in place, leaving the urine to sit all night. All I had to do was request that Gordon does not use the stopper and lets the fluid go down the drain.

This Gordon was willing to do. In his case, dementia didn't seem to prevent him from remembering the caregiver's instruction. Once I made my request, he was glad he could contribute to my well-being. And what a change that made in my judgment of him! I no longer thought of him as inconsiderate, but instead I perceived him as cooperative and caring.

Gordon had no problems with urine in the sink, nor all over the floor. It was I who had the problem. And I was contributing to the problem by judging him for his habit. I've learned to appreciate how I, the caregiver, contribute, and in a sense co-create "the problem," even though I do not have dementia.

We all are set in our ways, bound by social norms and personal habits. And through this lens we add to what we see as the *problem* in our own way. We contribute by blaming and judging the other person and by denying personal responsibility for our connection, for the relationship we both have with each other.

Must the problem be about me or them, exclusively? When the subject matter is caregiving, perhaps one could say that every problem is ours, in the sense that it affects our relationship, the way we are together. Dementia affects our relationship, and since one needs two to tango, we are both affected—we are both dealing with it. Difficulties associated with dementia, as Kitwood suggested, are located in the interpersonal. There is you, and there is the other person. But there is also your relationship.

Rumi, a Sufi mystic and poet, pointed out: "You think because you understand 'one' you must also understand 'two,' because one and one make two. But you must also understand 'and.'" The problem with dementia isn't necessarily in any one of us, per se: it is in the "and." It is in the way we relate to one another, in our relationship. Hence the answer is to be looked for "between" us. An ability to see this clearly, to own the difficulties that are associated with dementia, is a steppingstone in building a more satisfying relationship for both parties. Because dementia always affects more than the person who has been diagnosed with the condition.

When you take into account both the person and their dementia, yourself, and the relationship between you two—there is a dementia relationship.

Like any relationship, whether it is romantic, family, or professional, each dementia relationship is one of a kind. It may overlap with other types of relationships when it is a beloved, a relative, or a business partner who has dementia. Nonetheless, the dementia relationship requires us to make adjustments and establish new boundaries—as if we were running a family business or entering a working relationship with a spouse. We relate to each other according to context, to where and who we are, whether we are at home or at the workplace. In this case, we need to relate to each other while taking the context of dementia into account. Dementia will affect both parties in the relationship, perhaps in different ways, and to greater or lesser degrees, but nonetheless every person in a dementia relationship will be influenced in some way.

Dementia manifests in individuals so differently, one could almost say that dementia is custom-made, one of a kind. Each person differs both in their emotional reaction to the diagnosis and in the symptoms of their illness. Dementia can have a hugely varied range of symptoms, because it can affect different functions of the brain—language, memory, mobility, orientation in time and space, and perception. Whenever a caregiver turned over care of a client to me, I asked this crucial question: How does dementia affect this particular person? There are so many symptoms that one may not identify immediately. My intention is always to assume someone has their full capacity, and to support their independence as much as possible. Unless I had spent time with them before, I can't know whether someone is safe on their own. I can't know whether they can see accurately, whether what they see is real or part of their world only, or whether they know their limits and current capacities.

My next questions were: How does the illness affect the people around the person with dementia? How do they react to the symptoms? Which do they find challenging? Will I be able to sleep at night? Can I trust they will be okay making themselves a cup of coffee?

I asked these questions because dementia affects both parties. Dementia is a condition that two people share, even though only one may be carrying the symptoms of the illness. Yet we share its impact on our lives. Both of us must build a new relationship, with dementia in the picture. This is what I call a dementia relationship: it is *us*, with and without dementia.

Marshall B. Rosenberg said that "our survival as a species depends on our ability to recognize that our well-being and the well-being of others are one and the same." The well-being of a relationship affects two beings. A relationship can serve, nourish, and enrich. Relationships that are strong enough and occur between two connected individuals can be literally a survival strategy. Relationships can protect what's precious and human about us.

Humans as sentient beings have the capacity to feel, perceive, know and understand, respond, react, and be aware. Dementia affects all of these capacities, and hence it affects a person's state of being. I believe that it does not predetermine whether we experience well-being or ill-being, though. Ill-ness does not automatically imply ill-being. Rather, the state of our being is an indicator of our connection with other human beings.

Ill-ness does not automatically imply ill-being.

JUDGMENTS THAT BREAK RELATIONSHIP

The way we relate to one another can be empowering, or equally, it can be weakening. The more I bought into disconnecting thoughts and judgments, as if they were facts about the other person, the further away I was from the real them. Instead I was dealing with their caricature, a poor representation of the person who was in a dementia relationship with me.

This kind of thinking caused me suffering whenever Dory inquired about her concert tickets.

"Dear, we need to buy tickets for the performance this weekend. Good job, I just remembered! As usual, no one cared to remind me," Dory would say.

"No worries, Dory. I got the tickets for us already."

"Why didn't you tell me? Why did you keep it from me? It's only fair that I should know."

Inside, I felt rather aggrieved. Why does she always assume it was me who did something wrong? Why can't she see the fault in herself for once?

Feelings of hopelessness overcame me. What was the point? What was the point of telling her I'd already told her about the tickets three times? What was the point of reminding her about the tickets in the first place, as she would certainly forget to buy them herself? Then she would be annoyed that I didn't buy them for her. This went around and around in circles. Whichever way I went, whatever clever solution I came up with, we both lost. We both ended up disconnected.

What prevented us from connecting wasn't the tickets or the lack of memory, but the assumptions and judgments. It was each of us assuming that someone was wrong and to be blamed. Dory assumed I was mean and either hadn't reminded her about the tickets or had bought them behind her back. I thought she was unfair for always accusing me of bad intentions. I thought she was difficult or—in a more sophisticated form of blame that pretends it isn't blame at all—that it was her dementia that was difficult.

I was denying both my own and Dory's responsibility for the way we related to each other.

When we blame or accuse the other person of blaming us, we end up judging each other, which prevents connection from taking place. We disable our relationship. We fall out and our relationship becomes fragmented and disconnected. Each person in a relationship may be both contributing to this disconnection and be affected by it. It is a vicious circle which, once set in motion, carries on by force of habit. Was it the disconnection that came first and caused us to start blaming and judging each other? Or was it our blameful accusations that caused us to end up disconnected? Like with the chicken and the egg, we may never know which came first.

Dory and I habitually fell out over the purchase of her concert tickets and other arrangements that slipped her mind. For her part, I suspect she mistrusted my intentions.

This suspicion and distrust isn't uncommon among those living with dementia, and it doesn't come from nowhere. They have perfectly good reasons to be worried. The scenarios may differ from one person to the next, but from their point of view, some very suspicious things have been happening: a kettle has set itself on fire, their dressing gown turns up in the car, the parakeet is found motionless in its cage. From the perspective of the person with dementia, something isn't right.

As far as they are concerned, they had nothing to do with any of it, because they have no recollection of how these things came about. So it must be the fault of someone else—the spouse, the caregiver, the child, the neighbor. They might think: You are doing all of this deliberately to make me look stupid. You're plotting behind my back. And what the heck have you done to my parakeet!

Those on the outside may be blamed, judged to be wicked and insensitive, and labeled a bad husband, stupid caregiver, uncaring son, or vicious neighbor.

Whatever may be happening, the person with dementia has an underlying intuition that it is not good. Something is wrong. And whenever something is wrong, we tend to blame someone or something for it.

A person with dementia may judge themselves as the problem, rather than mistrusting others. They might think, I've become worthless now! They might turn against themselves, assuming that life is not worth living if one is not in full command of one's memory. Such self-judgment can have truly devastating effects. It can kill. The downward spiral of this thought pattern can lead people to contemplate suicide . . . until they forget all about it again. Ironically, this is how memory loss can save lives.

The worries never end, and they are just as concerning for those who care for someone with dementia: There is almost a fire in the house because an electric kettle is on the gas stove. Someone loses their way home at one in the morning after getting into the car to drive around in the middle of the night. They can't find the bathroom door, or forget how to open it, so they urinate by the wall. They stop feeding their parakeet, and it dies. And on top of it all, they forget your name. Again.

It's very easy to feel disconnected from someone judged as "making trouble" or "not trying hard enough." As if they are careless or insensitive. Because how else can we explain their behavior? Then one day we have a diagnosis, and we have a convenient label: dementia is to be blamed for all of it. We might say, Dementia has eaten up their brain, but what can I do about it? Yet we can take personal responsibility for the connection within our relationship.

The question is how do we take responsibility without blaming *someone* or *something*? We often assume that taking responsibility means also taking the blame. And then on one of those difficult nights, we may find ourselves absorbing the blame for not being patient enough, loving enough, skillful enough, understanding enough, foreseeing, preventing, or protective enough. Always falling short of "enough." No matter how much time we devote to caregiving, how much training we've done, how many self-help books we've read, and how many arrangements we've put in place to deal with this *problem*, during sleepless nights this sense of inadequacy and hopelessness may haunt us.

Self-criticism is as much a sign of disconnection as finding fault with someone else. Whether we judge ourselves or the other person is utterly irrelevant in this context. Both people in a dementia relationship can contribute to the disintegration of the relationship by blaming, judging, labeling, and denying responsibility.

ATTITUDES THAT DISABLE CONNECTION

Blaming: You plot behind my back. I'm not patient enough.
Judging: You're a bad husband. I'm such a horrible son.
Labeling: Dementia sufferer. Thickheaded caregiver.
Denying responsibility: The wretched illness has stolen my wife. This marriage is over.

When I was caught and imprisoned in this way of thinking, I saw Dory as lacking understanding. I saw her as failing, because she was unable to recognize that she had forgotten about the concert tickets. I saw my role as someone who had to be forgiving and to endure her deficits. In my mind, she was incomplete and incapable—that's why she needed me as her caregiver.

In conversations I had with her friends and other caregivers, we often discussed what Dory was losing, how her illness had progressed, and how there was less and less of Dory. "She's deteriorated since you were last here," I was told on a return to my caregiving role after a break.

It's no wonder we think this way. When our view of the person becomes all about their illness, we end up discussing the dementia more often than we discuss the actual person who has it.

Oliver Sacks has said that "neurology's favorite term is 'deficit,' denoting an impairment or incapacity of neurological function: loss of speech, loss of language, loss of memory, loss of vision, loss of dexterity, loss of identity, and a myriad of other lacks and losses of specific functions (or faculties). Everything that patients aren't and nothing that they are."

I am not a neurologist, but don't we all at times get fixated on what's wrong with someone? And we forget all about what's wholesome in them? We even do it to ourselves—though not diagnosed with any brain disease, we can still see all sorts of lacks and shortcomings in ourselves. With Dory, I saw myself as falling short of being patient and tolerant, not because of any neurological dysfunction but because, as I told myself, I wasn't a good enough person. There was never enough patience, care, time . . .

This scarcity perspective—thinking that there isn't enough of something or that we are lacking in quality—is equally limited. It contributes only to a sense of inadequacy. Caregivers of people with dementia are frequently reported to be at high risk for deterioration of their own mental health. And often the support that is available for caregivers, if any, focuses on troubleshooting specific symptoms, such as high blood pressure or an eating disorder. When caregivers get stressed or burned out, they are given medication or encouraged to develop coping mechanisms. Addressing the problem by tackling the physical and mental symptoms is one way that can help, but caregivers can also do something for themselves that is far more fundamental. They can focus on well-being by taking a bigger perspective. A new perspective can help them develop wellness through reconnecting with the person they care for.

As the American psychologists Christopher Peterson and Martin Seligman point out: "When psychiatrists and psychologists talk about mental health, wellness, or well-being, they mean little more than the absence of disease, distress, and disorder. It is as if falling short of diagnostic criteria should be the goal for which we all should strive."

Instead of striving for the absence of disease or illness, we could be striving for well-being—which is not an absence of illness or disability but actual fulfillment. Feeling fulfilled and satisfied is how well-being is experienced. It doesn't mean we will be happy ever after, but that we are feeling strong enough to face anything that life puts in front of us, including illness or disability, and that we can turn it into something that brings us together.

By contrast, when we focus on lacking capacity—such as not remembering, not being patient, not comprehending, or not being able to cope—and other potential flaws and faults of the cared for and the caregiver, both parties end up disconnected and dissatisfied. So even when there's only one person with an illness, when the relationship becomes ill, both people are, in a sense, unwell.

When we are stuck on ill-being, we focus on what we can't do or can't have. On the other hand, changing our perspective to focus on well-being enables us to see all the things we can do: the little skills, the things we like, the small bites of knowledge. These are the kinds of fundamentals we share as humans, regardless of our individual level of neurological fitness.

People with dementia can still laugh at a joke, dislike olives, be nutty about chocolate, cry over a broken cup, and admire a sunset. And through all of this, they can fulfill their need for fun and companionship, choice, pleasure, security, and beauty. And I say whoever can play, cry, or laugh wholeheartedly is whole.

A VISION OF WHOLENESS

When we adopt a bigger perspective, and we find ourselves in the bigger picture rather than losing ourselves in a list of lacks and losses, a whole new chapter in dementia relationship can open to us. Everyday life with dementia may appear lacking, impoverished, and incomplete, but it's a matter of how much light we are shining on the whole picture.

Someone with dementia, like Dory, who can't remember whether she bought the concert tickets, may appear lacking and incapable. Especially when she tried to make *me* responsible for any inconvenience her lack of memory caused. At the time, I heard blame. I saw Dory as incapable and confused, and I was resentful at not being trusted. Seeing things this way made us both miserable and grim. It felt like a dead end. When we feel stuck, we don't see things clearly, which is a sign that we're not recognizing things for what they really are.

But what happens when we, metaphorically, shine more light on the situation? Expand our narrow perspective? For example, look at this drawing.

Can you tell what it is? A tunnel with no light at the end of it? A black hole?

It's rather hard to tell. Let me shed some light on it.

This is the same drawing, except now you can see it more clearly.

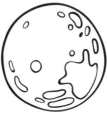

It is a moon.

The difference between them is that the first drawing depicts a new moon, an astronomical object in darkness, whereas the second picture depicts a full moon, the same object but fully illuminated. The first drawing looks like a hole, but in fact a whole moon is there. They're different phases of the same thing, with more or less light applied.

I once saw a cartoon that made a similar point. It showed the new moon walking into the doctor's office and saying, "I feel so empty." The doctor responded, "Don't worry, it's just a phase."

Like this new moon, Dory was only seemingly flawed. Despite her dementia, she had not lost her sense of fairness, and she cared about being included in the process of buying her concert tickets. She was afraid of being excluded, because it mattered so much to her to be seen and acknowledged. How can someone who cares so much be said to have lost their mind? What does it mean to say that she's not really there? As far as Dory was concerned, she certainly was very much there, with her needs and values that were alive for her, despite her dementia. Don't we all care about being acknowledged and taken into consideration?

Everyone, with or without dementia, has these universal needs. They are needs because we all need them for our well-being. They are also values because we value them in ourselves and others. They are principles because they are fundamental to who we are. And they are qualities because we can embody them in our actions and the way we express ourselves. Nonviolent Communication puts all wholesome human values, principles, and qualities under one umbrella name: universal human needs.

Universal human needs include connection, acceptance, affection, appreciation, belonging, respect, safety, trust, warmth, honesty, humor, celebration, beauty, ease, inspiration, order, autonomy, choice, challenge, clarity, competence, and more.

> connection,
> acceptance,
> affection, appreciation,
> belonging, compassion,
> consideration, inclusion, intimacy,
> love, mutuality, nurturing, respect/self-
> respect, safety, security, stability, support,
> to know and be known, trust, warmth, sexual
> expression, honesty, authenticity, integrity,
> presence, joy, humor, celebration, peace,
> beauty, communion, ease, equality,
> harmony, inspiration, order, autonomy,
> choice, freedom, independence,
> space, spontaneity, challenge,
> clarity, competence,
> consciousness

We value qualities such as these because they make our lives brighter.

Sometimes we feel that someone is lacking in certain qualities, not living up to certain values, or not fulfilling certain needs. Sometimes we ourselves feel like the new moon from the cartoon: empty, downhearted, and lacking. We can identify with this hollow state, as if that is who we really are in our core. But how we choose to view ourselves depends on our perspective—how we position ourselves in relation to the sun, and how much light, or attention, we shine on our world.

Regardless of whether we feel empty or full, we do continue to care. At least deep down. These universal human needs matter to us. The very longing of the new moon to be full again is a sign that those needs are hidden and unattended to, but not absent. We can strive to fulfill our needs, to shine the light of our attention on ourselves or others like the new moon, to reveal our wholeness, and to recognize our wholesome needs and values. Because when our needs are fulfilled, we feel like the full moon: glowing and full of radiance.

On days when I was able to hold this perspective, I never heard Dory complain. I never heard an accusation, and I didn't feel blamed for anything. In whatever words she used, I understood her to be expressing her needs. I heard how much she cared about being part of it all when she said things like "You bought those tickets without even telling me." Hearing someone say (or imply underneath it all) that they care about the same things we do is connecting. It brings us together. I find this perspective much more fulfilling than fixating on accusations. By bringing her needs to my attention, Dory was enriching our relationship with these qualities. Calling for our needs or values is like a call for life, for growth and maturity.

Originally I was missing trust and wanting Dory to have more faith in me. When I became aware that trust was what I cared about, I was able to become more trusting myself. I trusted that in her heart of hearts, Dory simply wanted her needs to matter too. We can embody the very things we wish for, and that's how we light up the darkness. Seeing ourselves and others in light of universal human needs makes connection inevitable—this was Marshall B. Rosenberg's message to the world.

Rosenberg's principles of Nonviolent Communication help us focus on what we value and find meaningful. They offer a bigger perspective on how to enrich one another's lives by discovering what motivates us, and what needs we are striving to fulfill. By illuminating our needs, we highlight their positive value. In relating to those with dementia, we can focus on skills they have and qualities they display, always striving to assume their wholeness.

We long for a sense of fullness and completeness that makes life worth living. It also makes life worth sharing.

All of us long for this full-moon sense of fullness and completeness that makes life worth living. It also makes life worth sharing.

COMPASSIONATE PARTNERSHIP

Sharing a life with someone who has dementia can enrich your life as well as theirs. People with dementia have full capacity to contribute to our well-being, or to our misery, depending on which perspective we have.

When our perspective is narrow, we generally don't see a person with dementia as someone worth sharing our lives with. I have witnessed many embarrassed, confused, uncomfortable, and at times horrified looks on the faces of people who simply did not know how to engage with someone who has dementia. People generally try to be sympathetic, and nice enough, but they also try to escape as soon as possible. Like I did with my great-grandmother. I left because I didn't know how to relate to her repetitive comments and confused statements. And I'm not alone. Many family members of people with dementia distance themselves, not because they don't care but because they don't know how to relate. I saw my clients' long-awaited visits from family turn into quick, fifteen-minute drop-ins. And the less a family member was able to relate, the greater the distance that grew between the relatives. Even close relatives can become strangers to one another over time.

On the other hand, the more connection we have in a relationship, the less we find differences in each other. We are able to see the person, with all their intact qualities, hidden behind the dementia. If we insist on perceiving a person through what their brains *can't* do, and evaluating them based on cognitive performance only, we may become so fixed on what *isn't* there that we miss altogether what *is* there.

If we become used to talking about and hearing about dementia in the context of suffering, damage, and misery, we will become used to thinking of those who have dementia as helpless, pitiful victims. We are unlikely to see "dementia victims" and "those suffering from dementia" as people with whom we can be in partnership. We will feel sorry for them, endure their company, and pass them by.

These expressions generate pity, not compassion. When we feel pity in a relationship, we categorize one person as pitiful, weak, and somewhat lacking, while in contrast the other person appears capable and "knows better." This sets up a dynamic of patronizing and infantilizing attitudes toward those with dementia, and that only makes our disconnection worse. This dynamic increases the feeling of dependency on the part of the person "suffering" and, in turn, increases the burden felt by the "capable" one, if they come to feel that all responsibility is now on their shoulders.

In these scenarios, those of us who have full mental capacity may experience a sense of having power over those who don't. This often comes with a sense of duty toward the other person, and feeling accountable for their health and physical condition. It's easy to put all that power and responsibility into making sure the person with dementia is in good physical condition—meanwhile, we forget to relate to them and to share the power we both have to make the relationship meaningful. This is another way to treat a person with dementia as pitiful, disabled, and lacking.

Pity is disengaging. People who pity others may attend a fundraising event or donate to a charity, but often they don't pay attention to those they are trying to support. In contrast, compassion is about togetherness. And it comes at a cost: it costs the value of our presence and empathy. Attention and presence are the most expensive, luxurious gifts we can give one another. Even though they don't cost money; they save so much of it! Engaging with another person in partnership not only provides a sense of togetherness, it can heal common symptoms of dementia such as emotional distress and challenging behavior. A content and connected dementia relationship can save nerves, time, and money—all needed to manage the many distressing situations in dementia care. Teaming up with the person you care for will make you both stronger, and you can share the power of your relationship.

But if we don't see someone as a partner, we won't know how to engage with them honestly. Pema Chödrön, author of *The Places That Scare You: A Guide to Fearlessness in Difficult Times*, puts it in the following words: "Compassion is not a relationship between the healer and the wounded. It's a relationship between equals. . . . Compassion becomes real when we recognize our shared humanity."

So calling someone a "dementia sufferer" or saying that someone is "suffering from dementia" harms the relationship by bringing pity and power inequality into play. These are highly inadequate expressions for several other reasons as well. First, none of the medical conditions that fall under the umbrella term *dementia* cause physical pain or emotional hurt for the person with the condition. Second, some people with dementia live well without suffering. The "suffering" that ensues may belong more to the relatives, friends, and care providers than to the person who has dementia. Finally, people with dementia do not want to be described as suffering. "Nothing about us without us" is a message they want people like you and me to understand. Let's not talk about them as if they can't enjoy life and personal power.

One summer when I was staying with Yvonne, her house was undergoing some (very necessary) work on the roof. That meant the house was wrapped in a net of scaffolding, and every now and then, workers' heads popped up through the windows. The family had warned the workers that it was better to stay out of Yvonne's sight, but she was rather observant. Besides, how can you hide scaffolding from the eyes of a house dweller?

As it happened, Yvonne was unnerved every time she discovered, to her great astonishment, the scaffolding and the people on it. What were these people doing climbing around her private house as they pleased?

Despite being told about the work on the roof, and having it explained to her on several occasions, Yvonne's agitation was stimulated again and again whenever she rediscovered the strange happenings outside her house. One day she decided to put an end to it, and she requested that I take her in her wheelchair to speak to these unwelcome guests. Which I did. A couple of workers, a woman and a man, stood there utterly frozen in confusion when Yvonne, firmly and definitively, told them off for intruding on her private property and demanding that they should all leave at once. She shouted, in her slightly throaty voice, "I wish to not see you again! You are to go away as soon as you get this ugly construction of yours from my house!"

The workers did not know what to do, or what to say. As far as they were concerned, they were hired to do a job, which they were dutifully doing. They did not respond to Yvonne's words at all, but she didn't care. I got her back into the house, and she appeared to be very pleased. "Now I've told them!" she said. I do believe that as far as she was concerned, her need to stand up for herself and to be heard was utterly fulfilled.

In a conversation later that day, I realized she did not in actuality want the workers to stop. It was true that she did not understand the necessity of it, but that wasn't what troubled her. It turned out that she wanted to be acknowledged as the owner of the house. To be seen and respected. In the end, she didn't care about the wretched scaffolding.

I went back briefly to explain to the workers about Yvonne's condition, and I told them what I had learned mattered to her. In response, I heard, "Poor lady." They felt pity for her.

This response was inadequate to Yvonne's situation. She wasn't "poor" in any sense of the word. She wasn't suffering, for a start— her health at that stage was pretty good. In terms of her finances, she was living comfortably. Moreover, Yvonne was decidedly not miserable; she was quite pleased with herself that she had told the workers off!

We requested that the workers report to her periodically to explain what they were doing in and around her house. She wasn't quite able to comprehend what was being explained to her, but again, that wasn't what mattered. Being acknowledged mattered. After being acknowledged, despite that she regularly forgot what the scaffolding was doing on her house, as if she had never seen it before, she remained much more settled in her emotional reaction to it. The workers' reports seemed to have truly met her need for recognition.

The fact that Yvonne had needs for recognition and acknowledgment did not make her weak or needy. Expressing her needs was an act of independence that showed how much personal power she was still holding, and that she was not letting it go. Her awareness of the needs and values she cared about had made her stronger and more empowered.

To dissolve the fake division between the "poor sufferers" and the "normal," we need to consider that dementia affects both parties in a dementia relationship. At times a relative, friend, or caregiver may carry a much heavier burden; they may suffer more than the person with dementia suffers. The person with dementia may be having a good time and feel more content and satisfied with themselves than ever before—which is to be celebrated. At the same time it is important to realize that a happy person with dementia does not necessarily result in a happy dementia relationship. The caregiving spouse, family member, or friend may still be strained. They may still experience overload, overwhelm, and overburden—emotionally, physically, financially, socially, or on several levels at once. This feeling of overload may not be understood by the person they care for, as people with dementia often release themselves from all responsibility for shopping, cleaning, personal care, or feeding.

A happy person with dementia does not necessarily result in a happy dementia relationship.

Thus dementia has an indirect effect on the caregivers of those who are directly affected. The needs of both parties have to be taken into account to build a genuinely fulfilling dementia relationship.

Dementia by itself is not a cause of suffering. Rather, the suffering, or ill-being, is the result of unfulfilled needs—often needs that nobody is aware of. A person's ability to adequately meet their own needs may be affected, even severely affected, by the disease. But the physical or mental condition of the brain on its own is never the sole cause of unhappiness.

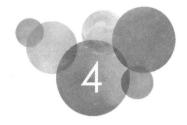

4

Committing to Life

To know life is to know intimately what you are feeling.
... It enables us to watch with mercy, if not humor, the
uninvited swirl of "mixed emotions" not as something
in need of judgment but as a work in progress.

—STEPHEN LEVINE, *American poet*

have heard people describe dementia using phrases such as "living death," "deadly disease," or "life sentence." Such phrases are not only incorrect, they fail to set us up well for a meaningful life. Such language prevents us from even recognizing the very real possibility of living well with dementia. And it simply denies what is happening all around the world—that people are realizing they can live fully, or at least meaning-fully, regardless of the condition of their brain.

What we need is language that enriches life instead of denying it. Marshall B. Rosenberg called this language Nonviolent Communication. The opposite of violence is peace. Nonviolent Communication is that which brings about peace, and restores connection. It is language that resurrects human connection from deadly disconnection, heals our sense of separation, and brings us back to life. That's why it is called the language of life.

A LANGUAGE OF LIFE

From the moment we are born, we are continually in the process of keeping ourselves alive. We do it by looking after our needs and fulfilling our values. There is no discontinuity between keeping our bodily needs met and keeping our existential needs fulfilled. A healthy body gives us a physical sense of aliveness, and satisfied values make us feel alive in another sense.

We do what life calls us to do, and when we are not meeting our needs, neither do we rest. We wriggle. When we need to go to the toilet, we wriggle physically. In much the same way, we wriggle internally when a need for respect or inclusion is not being met.

So we wriggle when we are lacking something, and we sigh in relief or joy when we have met a need.

Our human emotions range from the agony of unmet needs to the enjoyment of fulfilled needs. Our feelings are caused by the longings or fulfillments of our hearts. When we satisfy our needs, we feel comfortable. We feel full, or fulfilled. We feel like a full moon: hopeful, joyful, peaceful or thankful.

HOPE-FUL

absorbed, alert, curious, confident, empowered, enchanted, encouraged, energetic, engaged, engrossed, enthusiastic, entranced, expectant, fascinated, inspired, interested, intrigued, involved, optimistic, open, spellbound, stimulated...

JOY-FUL

amazed, amused, animated, ardent, aroused, astonished, awed, dazzled, delighted, eager, ecstatic, enthralled, excited, exhilarated, giddy, happy, invigorated, jubilant, lively, passionate, pleased, radiant, rapturous, surprised, thrilled, tickled, vibrant...

PEACE-FUL

blissful, calm, clearheaded, comfortable, content, enlivened, equanimous, fulfilled, mellow, quiet, relaxed, relieved, rested, restored, revived, satisfied, safe, secure, serene, still, tranquil...

THANK-FUL

affectionate, appreciative, compassionate, friendly, grateful, heartened, loving, moved, openhearted, proud, sympathetic, tender, touched, trusting, warm...

Conversely, when we are not meeting our needs, we feel dissatisfied and uncomfortable. Like the new moon from the cartoon I told you about earlier, we feel empty: disheartened, disquieted, displeased, disconnected.

DIS-CONNECTED

alienated, apathetic, ashamed, bored, cold, dejected, distant, fatigued, flustered, gloomy, guilty, hopeless, indifferent, lonely, numb, remorseful, sad, self-conscious, uninterested, withdrawn...

DIS-HEARTENED

anguished, bereaved, dejected, depressed, devastated, exhausted, gloomy, heartbroken, hopeless, hurt, lethargic, listless, melancholy, sleepy, tired, unhappy, worn out...

DIS-PLEASED

angry, appalled, contemptuous, disgusted, disgruntled, dismayed, enraged, exasperated, frustrated, hateful, horrified, impatient, incensed, livid, reluctant, resentful, spiteful, vexed...

DIS-QUIETED

alarmed, agitated, anxious, disconcerted, disturbed, frightened, mistrustful, panicked, perturbed, scared, startled, suspicious, terrified, troubled, uneasy, unnerved, upset, wary, worried...

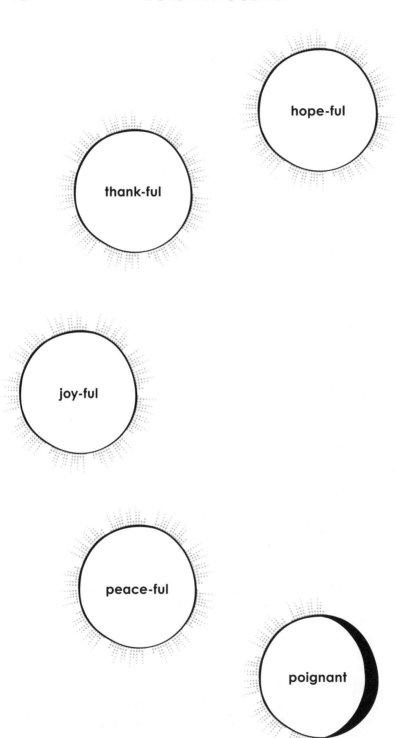

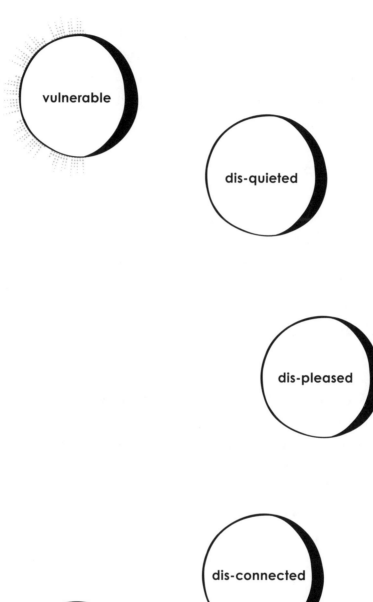
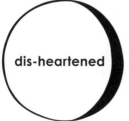

vulnerable

dis-quieted

dis-pleased

dis-connected

dis-heartened

If we feel dead, frozen, or numb, even this is still a sign of life. Because we always have feelings and always have needs. We may at times think that we feel nothing, and for some reason we think this is good because it protects us from hurt. But feeling nothing is simply remaining unaware of the life within us, which carries on regardless of our notice or approval. Feeling nothing is something we will not experience during our lifetime.

The more you allow yourself to feel, both physically and emotionally, the more you begin to see the connections between your deepest longings and your emotions, according to Sarah Peyton, a certified trainer with the Center for Nonviolent Communication and the author of *Your Resonant Self.* In other words, to discover the wholesome qualities we have deep inside, we have to be able to feel our emotions. Those emotions, those feelings, are indicators of what is and isn't fulfilled in us.

When I thought Dory was accusing me of plotting behind her back, I felt irritated because I longed to be trusted. I realized that trust, in this situation, was what mattered to me most. At first I saw this important value of mine as absent or missing—that trust didn't exist between Dory and me. But then I remembered the bigger perspective, the perspective of wholeness: that the entire moon is always there, even when some of it is in darkness. From this perspective, I could consciously choose to bring trust into our relationship—by embodying it, cherishing it, or asking Dory to have faith in my good intentions and to trust that her needs mattered to me.

There are many ways to move from the dark and empty phase of the moon into fulfillment. Whenever we shine the light of our awareness onto what's alive in us, whether those feelings are empty or satisfied, whether our needs are fulfilled or unmet, we can move toward more light and fulfillment. Like the moon moves out of shadow and into the sun. And when we are conscious of what it is that we need, we can judge our direction, and adjust accordingly. Like any living, sentient being would.

Tom Kitwood, author of *Dementia Reconsidered*, has devoted a lot of research to exploring indicators of ill-being among people who have dementia. He found that people with dementia show a lot of feeling, internal movement, or emotion. Unfortunately, that movement is often not toward life but rather away from it. Some people with dementia become withdrawn: they withdraw their attention and enthusiasm, and they become apathetic. Some seem to experience prolonged sadness and grief, causing them to lose interest in others and their surroundings and gradually become more disengaged and detached. Some demonstrate signs of boredom and hopelessness, whereas others seem to experience heightened states of agitation, anger, and despair.

But the dead don't experience despair. No matter how lifeless someone may appear on the outside, they are experiencing their own longing for fulfillment, or thirst for light, in their own way. If people with dementia were truly "gone," they wouldn't feel detached or disturbed. Instead, these noticeable emotions are indicators that point to the live needs which haven't been met. Nonviolent Communication, the language of life that focuses on needs, enables us to talk about this. Language which denies life, such as the language of neurological impairments and disabilities, only makes it harder for us to see the person behind dementia.

Language that denies life and the aliveness of needs leads many people straight to depression, or anger. Often, a diagnosis of dementia translates in people's minds into a death sentence, death that creeps slowly, taking each bit of self (such as memories, perceptions, and abilities) one by one. People with dementia may appear not very present, as if they were already gone. Even though they can still be found in their own homes, or in their residential care facility, they are not often visited. People without dementia sometimes say the places where those with dementia live are devoid of life. These people don't realize just how much they are ignoring. That in fact it is not life that is missing, but our sensitivity to it.

We are used to turning a blind eye to all the pain of unfulfilled needs, which is expressed quite openly by those with dementia, who are giving us obvious clues about the life within them.

People who ignore other people's expressions of life in the form of feelings—whether expressed directly or indirectly—generally do so because they are ignoring their own emotions. Once you learn to acknowledge your own feelings, you may discover that you share some of the very same feelings as the person you know who has dementia. Many people, with and without dementia, feel heartbroken and downhearted when the disease is identified. To some it means a terminal illness, and to others a burden of care. Hearts sink on all sides. It is common for people to feel distress so great that they blank out, disassociating themselves from their pain.

But when we disconnect our hearts, it is impossible for us to connect with someone. Connection takes place in the heart. Compassionate giving and empathic receiving flows to and from the heart, whether happy or in pain.

Using Nonviolent Communication as a language of life gives us a way to communicate that doesn't take away the pain, but makes that very pain sweet and enriching. This way of communicating connects us without shying away from the authenticity of the pain in our hearts.

A THOUSAND WAYS TO MEET NEEDS

It is not possible to make everyone happy at all times. Or if it is, I haven't learned it yet. But I do know it is possible to connect.

Finding ways into a meaningful relationship where everyone's needs matter is a realistic pursuit. However, most of us hold two unrealistic expectations about fulfilling our needs:

First, that meeting our needs means getting what we want.

Second, that the needs of two individuals in a relationship are, or are likely to be, in conflict.

Always getting what we want is impossible, which doesn't take long to figure out in the course of one's life. Because it may seem childish to hope for fulfillment of our longings, some people may give up on their needs altogether. This is especially true in a relationship in which our needs seem likely to bring disharmony. It would seem that a more reasonable, or compassionate, approach is to focus on someone else's needs, or to try to live up to someone else's values and principles.

Caregivers often hold strong beliefs that others' needs are more important than their own. This belief is usually acquired early in life if their direct expressions of need were met with discouragement or punishment. Believing that other people's needs are more important leads to not getting one's own needs met.

Marshall B. Rosenberg stresses that women often get the message early on that "to love" means "to give in":

> In a world where we're often judged harshly for identifying and revealing our needs, doing so can be very frightening. Women, in particular, are susceptible to criticism. For centuries, the image of the loving woman has been associated with sacrifice and the denial of one's own needs to take care of others. Because women are socialized to view the caregiving of others as their highest duty, they often learn to ignore their own needs.

It's easy for caregivers of any gender to see themselves as all about giving, even when they feel empty and depleted. As you strive to fulfill the needs of someone with dementia, consider how annoying a person who denies life in themselves can become! (Excuse my judgmental language.) I have certainly found myself complaining and moaning at times when I was unable to express my need clearly and directly. These strange behaviors seem designed to simultaneously disguise our needs and be obvious to another person, whom we expect to be able to read between the lines. We don't realize that by ignoring our needs in this way, instead of enriching others, we can make other people's lives miserable. Subconsciously, we are assigning someone else the responsibility for our unhappiness. Being in such a relationship is less than wonderful.

Going silent about what matters to you as a caregiver—simply shutting up—won't work either. You can only go so long without nourishing your needs before you will be burned out and flat on your face. This kind of relationship is not sustainable—it is more life-draining than sustaining. Denying our own needs, and trying to forget about things that matter to us, impoverishes the relationship. It leaves the relationship, and consequently the very person you are sacrificing yourself for, deprived of the values and qualities you could be contributing, if only you were able to listen to your needs.

To enrich each other, we need to bring our broader perspective to the dementia relationship. A broader perspective includes and sustains the needs of both the cared for and the caregiver. When we examine some of our needs and some of their needs, we discover that many of them are shared, like shared property in the relationship. These needs may include respect, warmth, understanding, safety, rest, and fun.

"There is one need missing on this list of needs," said a woman at one of my workshops, half-joking, after we read some of the universal human needs. "I've got a need for smoking that isn't listed here—yet I'm certain I have it!"

When I asked her what smoking gave her, I meant to direct her attention to what need of hers was being met by smoking. Smoking, like money or a house, is never a goal in itself. It is simply a strategy to give us something. Money can give us safety, and a house can fulfill a sense of belonging in us.

We tend to cling to our ideas of what will satisfy us because the need underneath is important. Certainly we get something out of smoking a cigarette, or having a nice sum of money in a bank account. When this woman and I started talking about the role smoking played in her life, it became obvious to both of us that it would be very difficult for her to give up smoking as long as she believed that smoking was her actual need.

She explained that, as a single mother, she looked after a disabled adult son, as well as two younger sons at home. Every day was full of the responsibilities of running a demanding household. She took her motherly duties very seriously, never complaining, but also never allowing herself a break . . . except for a cigarette. Going out for a cigarette guaranteed her time to breathe some air (tragic as that may sound) and, as she put it, "does her good." Her smoke breaks were her only blame-free downtime, the only time she had to look after herself. She was addicted to cigarettes because smoking was her way of meeting her needs for space, freedom, and relaxation.

You can see how important it was for her to continue this habit: without it, she wouldn't know how to access the feelings of relaxation and freedom without which her life would be hard to handle, even unbearable.

As we explored the difference between a need, such as freedom or relaxation, and a strategy, such as smoking, she became silent, and perhaps even a little irritable. It's never easy to see that the thing we cling to is not something we need, but is something we think we want, which may or may not be truly serving us. The woman at my workshop had a strategy that was trying to satisfy important needs. It was also leaving a cloud of smoke in her lungs. This realization was a sobering and perhaps uncomfortable experience.

The good news is that there are numerous ways to meet our human and commonly shared needs for space and freedom. Each of us does it in our own way.

I met the woman in my workshop some time later, and found to my delight that she had decided to get a dog with her sons. The dog required regular walks outdoors, which fulfilled her needs for space and freedom without compromising her needs for health and independence, both of which had not been well met by her addiction to smoking. She was able to meet her needs more accurately, and had therefore been able to overcome wants and urges that didn't serve her as fully.

When we commit to discovering our needs and taking them seriously, myriad possibilities open up before us. One of my Nonviolent Communication mentors, Kirsten Kristensen, likes to say there are a thousand ways to meet each and every one of our needs—as long as we are clear about the difference between the things we truly need and value, and the strategies we adopt to try to fulfill those needs.

Confusing *what* we need and *how* we fulfill that same need has serious (I mean serious) consequences for us.

When I say to myself, I'm worthless, I am not meeting my own need for acceptance, this self-talk becomes a self-defeating mechanism which disconnects me from my longing.

When someone goes out for a cigarette because she wants a breath of fresh air and freedom, she will get the opposite of what she really needs. When we go to war because we want peace, it is unlikely we will get what we truly long for.

Clearly distinguishing our needs from our wants and strategies is key. Choose strategies that do correspond and are likely to fulfill your longings and you will be able to help others do the same.

Dementia does not affect a person's needs and values. People, with or without dementia, need freedom, choice, safety, humor, and friend-ship. These needs can be the platform on which we build our relationships, an underlying thread that connects our hearts. In other words, needs can bring people together rather than set them apart.

Our needs can be the platform on which we build our relationships. They can bring people together rather than set them apart.

This brings us to the second false assumption: that the needs of two individuals in a relationship are, or are likely to be, in conflict.

Most of us are convinced that we cannot meet everyone's needs. This assumption traps us in an "either you or me" way of thinking. It leads caregivers to believe that our only two choices are to become a self-denying giver or a self-serving egotist. What an impossible choice!

Learning that there are many ways in which we can meet needs, without downplaying or denying any of them, serves all of us so much better. I wish I had known this when I was a young girl living with my own family all those years ago, because this knowledge can help with so many ordinary family dramas, not only those complicated by dementia.

My sister and I shared a room throughout our childhood

By acknowledging everyone's needs, you can escape the impossible choice of becoming either a self-denying giver or a self-serving egotist.

and early teenage years, and at the time, it was hard enough having two teenage girls under one roof, let alone in the same room. It was tough for our parents to witness our fights, but also for us, needing to perform all these grand dramas quite regularly. If only we'd had better communication skills, and more trust in the possibility that a win for one needn't be a loss for the other.

We regularly encountered conflict over our different needs during after-school hours. My sister enjoyed meeting her needs for fun and play by listening to MTV, newly available on television at that time, whereas I generally wanted to meet my needs for rest and space after the noisy school hours by resting quietly and reading a book. You might think these needs were obviously in conflict: her need for fun and entertainment, and my need for rest and space. We thought so too. And so we fought.

These fights were rather unimaginative ways to pursue what really mattered to us. And neither of us ended up meeting our needs: she did not meet her need for fun (having just heard many unpleasant adjectives directed toward her), and I certainly did not meet my need for rest. It was a lose-lose situation.

At the time, I wished she wasn't there. She was a problem! Everything would have been fine without her! And it had been fine, I thought—before she was born.

When I think about how I wished my sister had never been born, I am so relieved this wish was never granted. Stories tell us to be careful what we wish for. I say we need to be equally careful what strategies we choose to pursue to fulfill our wishes.

Trying to fulfill our needs without knowing our heart is pretty hopeless. The strategies we identify are often based on an inaccurate perception of the situation, which we arrive at through labeling and blaming everyone involved. Instead of choosing what served us most, we blindly choose

Different needs are never in conflict. They enrich the same life in different ways.

strategies that result in hurtful conflict and deadly disconnection. To open our eyes to the possibilities, we need to get to know our own hearts first.

If I had known in my heart that I simply needed rest (and not to annihilate my sister), then I could have come up with more imaginative solutions than picking a fight. I could have asked her to put headphones on while I took a nap. Or I could have gone into my parents' bedroom to rest after school, which I knew they did not mind. Or my sister could have gone into the living room to watch television. There were so many simple options we were oblivious to.

As an adult and a student of Nonviolent Communication, and as a caregiver to Dory, I was so much more aware of what was going on in my heart that eventually I became conscious of my own needs, and I was able to guess her needs too. I knew I was longing for trust, and I was pretty sure she greatly valued being included and taken into consideration. Still, coming up with a way to fulfill both of our needs required a few trial runs.

For example, we tried putting the concert tickets that she continually forgot about somewhere visible, like on Dory's coffee table, so that she would be reassured that the tickets had been purchased and had been brought to her attention. This solution worked for me too, temporarily, because Dory was thankful to have the tickets and no longer accused me of making plans behind her back. There they were—right in front of her! Until she decided to put them somewhere safe . . . never to be found again. So we needed a different strategy. In the end, we wrote up a notice, nice and clear, saying that the tickets had been reserved and paid for and would be collected before the concert. This solution relieved us both of mistrust and resentment and made our life together so much easier.

To see the bigger picture, we need the perspectives of both people in the relationship—the person with dementia and the caregiver. This creates greater chances of connection, for greater possibilities in a life with dementia—together.

Once we see the bigger picture, we're ready to learn the skills that will help keep us connected. This is what the rest of this book is about.

PART TWO

TASTING FOR YOURSELF

Caregiving can be a way to enrich your own life. You will find many ways to fulfill your needs, some inside and some outside of your caregiving role. When you acknowledge your own needs, you are in a better position to connect with other people.

HOW TO CONNECT WITH YOURSELF

- Make a habit of self-empathy, your emotional daily hygiene.
- Give yourself time to reflect, and find a convenient, private space for it.
- Stay up to date with your immediate sensations and feelings.
- *Feel* your feelings, don't *think* them.
- Learn to see all feelings as reminders that indicate met or unmet needs.
- Supercharge your inner power by attending to your own needs—through self-empathy or through interaction.

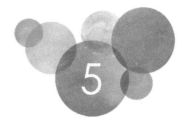

Cultivating Empathy

The reason we are often not there for others
is that we are not there for ourselves.

—PEMA CHÖDRÖN, *Buddhist author*

When you're traveling, you might ask your phone for directions. But no GPS can help get you there unless it knows your point A—your starting point. It is impossible to get anywhere unless you know your own location.

In the same way, you cannot connect with another person until you are connected with yourself. You, the person who cares for someone with dementia, are a necessary component in a satisfying dementia relationship. Connecting with another person does not mean merging with the other person to the extent that you are no longer there yourself. For a wholesome connection, you are needed as a distinct individual.

Therefore, don't forget to count yourself in your dementia relationship.

When my husband and I got married, we counted the number of wedding guests we expected and arranged for the right number of chairs. But shortly before the ceremony, someone pointed out that we had forgotten to include ourselves in the count, so we had two fewer chairs than we needed to seat everyone. This was easily dealt with at the time, but it made me realize how easy it is to forget about yourself, even at your own wedding. This chapter is about how to count yourself in. It is never too late to pull up another chair.

To be part of a dementia relationship means extending care to yourself. Nonviolent Communication gives us a process through which we can take care of ourselves fully—by becoming aware and responsive to the full spectrum of our feelings and needs, omitting none. The Nonviolent Communication practice of getting to know yourself better by feeling your feelings and sensing your needs is called self-empathy. The better I know and acknowledge myself, the more I become a connoisseur of connection. Tasting the sweetness of connection firsthand is arguably the best way to know it.

CARING FOR YOURSELF

Have you ever heard people justify not attending to their basic hygiene due to lack of time? I have been so busy this week, I didn't even brush my teeth for five days! Does anyone really say this?

I don't hear people making such comments but I do hear people say they don't find time to attend to their own feelings and needs. They do not have time for self-connection and emotional hygiene, or, in the language of Nonviolent Communication, for self-empathy.

Looking after yourself is not a selfish thing to do. You might think that ensuring empathic time for yourself is a private matter that doesn't concern anyone else, but it does: it affects everyone with whom you are in contact. Think about how your lack of bodily hygiene might affect those who are near you. Lack of heart hygiene will affect your nearest and dearest too. The way you are in yourself, how fulfilled you are, affects your capacity to communicate empathically with others. It also affects your imagination and your ability to come up with life-enriching strategies. Imagination is a sign of a resourceful mind and a heart that knows empathy.

Practicing self-empathy is an ongoing activity that, like brushing your teeth and keeping yourself clean, can become integrated into your daily routine.

PRACTICING SELF-EMPATHY

You can practice self-empathy anytime and anywhere, but I have found that taking a moment for myself, in quiet, helps me reconnect. I don't need to provide an excuse to look after my own needs, but sometimes it helps to stop the conversation or leave the room to give myself the space to reflect. There is another similarity between self-empathy and bodily personal hygiene: you can use the bathroom for both. I remember one time, Elizabeth English, my mentor in Nonviolent Communication, excused herself from the group she was leading for a toilet break. Afterward she told me that she had used this time to connect with herself, to give herself empathy: the bathroom provided a convenient private space to do so. Simple habits of coffee breaks, journeys on public transportation, or walks with a dog can also provide moments to reconnect.

Cultivating empathy for yourself on a daily basis is important because you are important. You are important in yourself, and you are important, vital, and necessary to the person you care for. Without you, no connection is possible. Who is there to connect with, if you are not there? Practicing self-empathy will anchor you to weather the rough storms that may come. And you will in turn be an anchor to others by connecting to the depths of your own heart.

Because you are the person with the most direct access to yourself, you are the person who can empathize with yourself most intimately, more than anyone else in the world. Paying attention to your inner life, and practicing self-empathy as I mentioned earlier, is one of the most effective ways to fulfill your needs. It is a powerful method of self-care. And it is safe to try at home, on your own.

In her book, *Your Resonant Self,* Sarah Peyton points out that when we are disconnected from our inner life, we may experience sudden outbursts of emotion that seem to come from nowhere.

When people are experiencing emotional upset but don't know it, pressure can gradually build over time, resulting in a sudden and seemingly inexplicable explosion into unregulated distress: unpredictable temper tantrums, black holes of despair, or uncontrollable sobbing. These people may feel like they are standing beside themselves, seeing their own desperation, and simultaneously unable to understand it.

You may find it hard to believe, but these emotional eruptions are healthy reactions: your organism is demanding self-care. In the practice of Nonviolent Communication, we learn to see all feelings as reminders, with information indicating met or unmet needs. Dis-ease can be a sign of dis-connection from yourself. Emotions don't come from nowhere. If you feel lost, it's because you've lost your bearings and don't quite know where you are, or where your inner "location" is.

I've known caregivers who experienced emotional breakdowns to the point where they could not continue looking after the person they cared for. Such a collapse is most likely preceded by long-unacknowledged feelings.

We all need to get to know ourselves better and become familiar with our inner land. This landscape will continue to surface, and if you get to know it and familiarize yourself with its topography, you can turn it into your playground. On the other hand, if you leave your inner land unexplored, it may appear scary and dangerous, with emotional traps all over the place.

So go and have a look within. Claim this place as your inner home. Look again. Sense within. Your heart's eye needs to get used to the inner environment for its vision to come back into focus. Like when you walk into a cellar and you need a moment for your vision to adjust to unlit space. After some time, you will start to notice things to see, emotions to feel, and needs to sense. That's the beginning of getting to know your inner space. Being empathic toward ourselves becomes possible only when we are familiar with our inner land. By claiming this land back from the unconscious and repressed, we claim our inner heritage back, and our life is enriched.

"But I don't know what to do" is a good place to start, because not knowing is an open state of mind. The first step is to get to know yourself a little, as if for the first time. Because you need to know yourself well enough to successfully attend to your own needs. Most of us have not been acquainted with ourselves much over the course of our lives. Hence we are not that familiar with our interiors. Perhaps we found a way in once and then got lost in the unfamiliar inner world of ours. Maybe we were overwhelmed by strong emotions accompanying a traumatic event or painful situation. Maybe we didn't know how to get out once we were in, and once we finally escaped, we kept the door closed ever after.

Or maybe we think of ourselves as the kind of person who is not emotional or "not good with feelings and that sort of stuff." Maybe we think feelings are irrational and could make us act impulsively and do things we might later regret. Maybe our inner life has become dominated by thinking, and thinking alone. We even *think* our feelings, because we never learned (or forgot) how to feel them, and the actual feelings, and other unwanted items, are kept in a cellar which we don't often visit. When we look within, we see nothing and assume there is nothing to see. If we genuinely do not sense what we are feeling, we really don't have a clue what we need. It's as if we are not up to date with our own inner events and happenings.

We think our feelings because we never learned (or we forgot) how to feel them.

To update your inner knowledge of yourself, become more interested in your most immediate sensations and feelings. Ask yourself: What am I sensing in my body? How am I feeling? The answer may not come with words, and that does not matter. What is important is your curiosity about your inner life. It may lead you to inquiring about your needs: What is it that I care about here? What do I want to do about it?

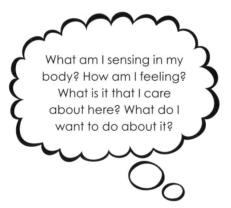

What am I sensing in my body? How am I feeling? What is it that I care about here? What do I want to do about it?

Remember, your dementia relationship needs both parties. Empathy for yourself is vital because it brings connection back to life.

When disconnection strikes, it may cause coldness, the rift of separation, or the heat of hurt and burning anger. When I cared for Gordon, his wife, Jenny, kept a cold distance from her husband. I suspect she feared that closeness or open conversation would bring out too much hot anger and resentment for her to bear. So when Gordon entered a room, Jenny left almost simultaneously, perhaps unconsciously. It seemed that the distance had to be kept because their orbits could no longer meet, and they were left in their own lonely trajectories around, but not with, each other. Years of emotional distance had created disconnection between this good-natured couple.

The untimely death of connection, when a relationship between two people withers and hearts disconnect, can be one of the greatest pains the human heart will ever experience. This pain, unlike physical pain, cannot be treated with pills and injections. The best diet in the world will not bring connection back to life. When the heart is closed, nothing gets in.

It is perhaps counterintuitive that in order to restore the sense of aliveness and connection in ourselves and with others, we need to turn to the very place that aches the most: our hearts. The heart can ache in various ways. Some people feel acute pain, while others feel nothing, which is another form of pain: the heart plays dead to avoid, disassociate, rationalize, and blank out—to feel nothing rather than feel the pain.

Does it sound like I'm talking about the disillusionment of romantic love or a love affair that ended tragically? Ask anyone who has been diagnosed with dementia, or ask their spouse or children, whether their hearts aren't aching. Ask yourself. Once the heart that's in pain closes and attempts to feel nothing, the connection is broken further.

Now, this may have happened for you well before dementia came into play. It does for many. Yet even if your heart has been "out of service" for some time now, the diagnosis of dementia probably triggered some pain, fear, or fury. The pain is not the worst thing that can happen to you. This pain of disconnection is your heartbeat. This trigger is your life spark, even at the precise

The pain of disconnection is your heartbeat.

moment that you may desperately want to close your heart, again, from experiencing the pain and from feeling vulnerable and open.

Vulnerability is an ability to be radically honest about how you really are, and it can become a real strength. We can become stronger and at ease with painful emotions because even though they hurt, they can't really harm us. These are feelings to be recognized for what they are and nothing more than that. They will point toward the longing of your heart.

Be who you are, no matter how you are. We often try to escape ourselves because we are not at home with who or how we are. But as has been said before, "Be yourself—everyone else is already taken." No one else can be you, no one else can fill your shoes.

Dis-comfort, or uneasy emotion, is a telltale sign of dis-connection. You may feel uncomfortable in your body, or you may feel pressure on your chest or tension in your muscles. You may be aware of nothing but your pain, in which case you already know you need some time for yourself, and right now. But sometimes you won't be aware of *how* you are at all. In that case, how do you know if you need time for yourself?

Most of us wake up to these signs when we are being shouted at by loud, judgmental thoughts. As soon as you spot any thoughts that judge your own or another person's worth, you know you need self-empathy. I might judge myself and my caregiving by thinking: I'm really rubbish at this, or I'm not good enough, or I should be more compassionate. I might also judge the other person. In my dementia relationship with Gordon, I noticed myself thinking, He always thinks women are here to serve him. That was a clear judgment to spot, and when I realized I was judging him, I knew straightaway that I was uneasy about something. And instead of building a story line of Gordon's chauvinism, I used it as a signpost to my own feelings and needs.

Admitting that we sometimes think such harsh things about the people we care for is hard for any caregiver, whether a paid professional or an unpaid relative. These judgments may at first seem like the opposite of love and care. But underneath each judgment are feelings that point right back at our own living needs and values, or qualities of consideration, care, and respect. If we ignore our judgmental thoughts, we risk throwing the baby out with the bath water—we may reject the feelings which indicate our met or unmet needs. Instead of rejection, we need to make time for self-empathy to learn what we need and what we can offer.

To start the process of self-empathy, identify your judgmental thinking, and instead of following that judgmental thought chain any further, redirect your attention to your body.

How are you now?

You may be able to register some troubling sensations, or you may spot tension in certain areas of your body. You may not. Maybe what you experience at the moment is only your mind crowded with thoughts, opinions, and all the things you would have or should have said.

Is what you experience cold or hot? Allow yourself to experience the temperature of your feeling—hot, cold, or somewhere in between. Cold feelings are often associated with sadness, loneliness, and isolation. Feelings that are fiery hot might be anger, irritation, and frustration. The comedian Steven Wright has been credited with saying that depression is anger without enthusiasm. Sometimes feelings seem to be more visible and insist on our attention, and sometimes they hide behind the back of mental states. Our job is not to put them right, but simply to acknowledge them.

Allow yourself to experience the temperature of your feeling, whatever it is. If all that comes to mind is, But I can't feel anything!—well, how does it feel to feel nothing? And it's okay to say that it just feels empty. Your feeling doesn't need a name to be acknowledged. Feelings, like children, seek attention. They like to be seen.

That is the true role of feelings: to attract your attention. You do not need to play with them before you acknowledge they are there. If your feelings are blank, and instead you experience lots of thoughts rushing through you, stop a moment and imagine how you might be feeling. Imagine how someone who is not you, but who is like you, might feel in your situation. What comes to your mind?

Feelings, like physical pain, play a very important role, which is to keep you informed. The only function of physical pain is to inform you that something within you isn't okay and requires attention. Feelings are informative in the same way: they point toward your needs. Something in your system is out of balance. You may have an idea straightaway what your feeling is about. You may think: I miss understanding or I long for appreciation. These feelings are signals that might relate to needs that are unmet, unfulfilled, or distant like dreams. Feelings of joy or contentment may be signals letting you know your needs have been fulfilled, when dreams come true.

The only purpose of physical pain is to inform you that something within you isn't okay and requires attention.

Whatever need is now demanding your attention, it existed already. It is part of you. It is your heart speaking to you. It is in your very nature to have needs, and to gravitate naturally toward fulfilling them—because once a need is fulfilled, it turns into one of the qualities of your being that makes you who you are. If I long for appreciation, that is because when I am being appreciated, when my need for appreciation is met, I am more myself. I am naturally kinder, more open, and more patient, without needing to put on a "good caregiver show" and contrive my behavior.

It is very hard to act kind, be open, and remain patient when our needs aren't fulfilled. On the other hand, when our needs *are* fulfilled, these qualities of kindness, openness, and patience come forth naturally, and—to our great relief—effortlessly. The only moment you will need some willpower is the moment you summon the courage to turn within and see what it is you are longing for.

I can understand why turning within to identify what you are longing for may be difficult for some people to do. If you have been motivating yourself by saying you have to do something because it is the right thing to do, then you may judge your feelings inside as a nuisance, or a weakness. You may think: I don't *feel like* doing all this, but it's what I have to do.

Notice that self-talk doesn't touch on what you are feeling. Are you fed up, burned out, or weary? Any of these emotions could point you toward something that is as important to you as the care that you are providing. And I'm here to tell you that whether your need is for inspiration, ease, fun, or anything else, acknowledging it will very likely strengthen your dedication to care rather than weaken it by making you "lazy" or "irresponsible." By connecting to your feelings and needs through self-empathy, you are making sure that you have the capacity to enrich someone else's life as well as your own.

We don't have to strive to be perfect at what we do, because we can find something life-enriching in our less-than-ideal experiences.

LIVING WITH IMPERFECTION

Some days I am not as patient as I wish I were. Some days I am less than perfect. Probably most days, if I am being honest. Some days you will also run out of inner power and will need to support yourself, and you may be unable to provide as much support to the other person in your dementia relationship. If these days coincide with the particularly confused days of the person you're caring for, there is little chance they will be able to provide empathic support to you. And if you spend extended time running low on resources and drawing on empathic reserves, both of you may end up in explosive anger. You need to be able to take care of yourself if you want to help others in meaningful and enjoyable ways.

I learned this lesson the hard way with Dory. One day she had just come back from visiting her best friend, Beth, who had lived with Alzheimer's for many years and now lived in an assisted living unit in an advanced stage of the illness. Dory found the visit with her friend very unsatisfactory. She said, "There's no point in going to see Beth anymore. She can't recognize me, she doesn't remember what we talked about last time, and she simply doesn't make any sense."

I heard her words and wondered whether Dory recognized her own confusion. But no, she appeared completely unaware that she and Beth shared the same illness. Dory thought of herself as "the normal, all-together one" as opposed to "the demented friend." She was annoyed with their pointless conversations, and she questioned whether Beth was even her friend anymore, given that their shared friendship history was forgotten. "Beth is gone. I think I shall stop visiting her. I'm just wasting my time," Dory said.

At first I was uneasy. As I continued listening to Dory, my unease and frustration soon rose to the heights of anger. The more I thought about what I heard, the more angry I felt. My mind was bombarded with thoughts like these: You selfish cow! You yourself forget things, sometimes on an hourly basis. And yet your friends stand by you no matter what. No matter how many times you forget their name, confuse them with someone else, or don't express yourself clearly. And what kind of friend are you to someone in exactly the same condition as yourself? You are selfish and ungrateful!

My judgment, in other words, was that she didn't deserve the support she got from her friends, because she herself was so ungrateful and mean. This judgment only fueled my anger further, but thankfully Dory's gardener came around. Her visit allowed me to take a walk on my own and leave Dory in the gardener's company.

I walked and talked to myself, not out loud, but my thoughts were written in angry red letters, and each exclamation point was followed by another, and then another shouting thought. The caricature of Dory in my head was the personification of everything I wanted to fight against, like an enemy image. Judgmental thoughts turn other people into simplistic caricatures. This was a sure sign that I needed some empathy, to heal the heat and pain of my anger. As I walked, I phoned my friends, who I could call anytime to share my troubles.

Judgmental thoughts turn other people into simplistic caricatures.

The first friend I called said, "You shouldn't blame Dory. It's this dreadful Alzheimer's that makes her say things like that."

The second friend said, "If you're going to take things so seriously, you won't last in this job. You just need to hold your breath and bear it."

The third friend said, "I know what you mean, I had a client like that once. What happened to me was . . . "

Each friend meant well. They tried to frame the problem intellectually, give advice, or sympathize. None of their advice spoke to my heart. I needed empathy.

Relying on empathy from others is not always possible, but this does not mean our need for connection has to remain unsatisfied. Sarah Peyton notes that human beings are wired for connection. And that this urge for connection is so fundamental to how we are built that our nervous system is capable of acting as our own compassionate self-witness. In self-empathy we use our own ears to listen to ourselves.

In self-empathy we use our own ears to listen to ourselves.

In this situation with Dory my heart needed to be heard. And I happened to have my own pair of ears, so I stopped and listened. I sensed tension when I remembered Dory's comment, and I felt anger when I recalled my thoughts about it. But when I allowed myself to feel what I felt, rather than think what I felt, or explain away what I felt, I heard loud longing. This longing was for kindness and consideration—two things I care deeply about. I also care about people with dementia being seen, understood, and included.

Ah, what a relief it was to recognize this! Yes, I care. These values—for kindness and consideration—are alive in me. And I can stand by them, right at the center of my being.

When we are crystal clear about our values and needs, everything becomes clearer. So when we experience empathy, we tend to say things like all is fine, all is okay, or all is good. And it does feel as if literally *everything* is okay. Being full of this feeling is fulfilling, like when the new moon turns into the full moon.

I wasn't able to see this until I paid attention to myself and myself alone. Until I had a moment to take a look inside, rather than jumping into solutions to correct others' behavior or my own.

Once I was at ease, I was able to see that Dory herself was expressing some pain. I could imagine she might have been feeling discouraged and sad, perhaps disappointed, when Beth didn't recognize her. Perhaps for Dory it was about her need for acknowledgment, connection, and friendship. Maybe she was expressing her longing for connection with Beth.

I brought the subject up during our supper that night, now that I was able to hear her. So it was worth paying attention to my own needs and cherished values first, because I was then at ease to open my heart to Dory again.

How *you* are matters greatly in a dementia relationship. You are an essential component to a satisfying relationship with someone affected by dementia. There is no way your relationship with the person who has dementia will flourish if you are not cultivating empathy and nurturing your inner power. You will need them both, believe me.

ASKING FOR EMPATHY OUT LOUD

There are times when I run out of inner power and choose to ask for empathy from the other person in my dementia relationship. Expressing a need for empathic understanding isn't a last resort, but expecting empathy from someone who has cognitive problems with comprehending what's going on around them—well, it may seem too optimistic. And yet, as I've learned from Clare, cognitive impairment does not affect the heart's ability to connect. It may just take bit of time.

One day as we approached Clare's dressing room, where I went every day to help her get dressed, I wondered how long it would take.

You wouldn't think it could take long, would you? There are clothes, there is Clare, there is a caregiver—me—and there is willingness in both of us to get dressed in an optimal amount of time. And yet every day the amount of time it took to get dressed was a lottery. We might be there ten, twenty, thirty, forty, fifty minutes, an hour, occasionally even longer. I called it "the dressing-room phenomenon," or "the hell of losing my patience." Various factors contributed to this little pocket of eternity in which we could be caught for a long, long time.

For a start, even though Clare was in her late eighties, she still took pride in what she wore—not only for comfort, but also for how she looked. Perhaps I had thought once a person reached a certain stage in life—as long as they were comfortable and clean—they ceased to care about their appearance. Well, that was certainly not true in Clare's case. Even if we planned to be home all day, with only each other as company, that made no difference to her choices about her appearance. It was about how she felt in whatever she was wearing and how she looked to herself in the mirror. Despite her severe sight impairment, and the regular examinations by orthoptic specialists trying to find ways to improve Clare's vision, when it came to examining her appearance in the mirror, Clare's eyesight was never mistaken. She spotted the slightest color imbalance or the tiniest speck of dirt. Her standards were outrageously high.

Another factor that played into the dressing-room phenomenon was that dementia had affected Clare's decision-making ability, but curiously, not her awareness of this disability. In other words, she believed she was capable of making decisions and so expected herself to choose correctly in accordance with her own needs.

Clare also had difficulty finding the right words to express what was on her mind. Often she struggled to describe a particular piece of clothing she was looking for. I joined in her search by trying to guess what she was after—using my imagination, you see. Sometimes I was successful in finding the right word, or even better, the right trousers, and yet even that didn't necessarily mean success in getting her dressed.

There also was a discrepancy between Clare's size and her self-image. She had gained weight considerably over the last few years before I met her, and certain clothes didn't fit her anymore. Unfortunately, many of her favorite dresses and trousers were now too small. Even if we found something she liked, something that she remembered being comfy and presentable, it didn't work because it no longer fit. Meanwhile, any new piece of clothing was looked at with suspicion. New trousers appeared far too big, even though they were the right size.

Clare was never aggressive. Yet after fifty minutes in the dressing room she became highly irritable. Eventually she sighed in resignation. It was a great big exasperated *sigh*, loaded with meaning. It seemed to say, Either you are an idiot incapable of putting some decent clothes on me, or I am the idiot myself . . . This assumed judgment is what I needed to translate empathically.

Initially I tried to take the lead by suggesting a simple solution—something I knew she liked. I focused on nice, warm, comfy, clean, fitting, and elegant clothing. I made sure to move other pieces of clothing out of sight, so as not to distract her. Occasionally, when we were in a rush—like when she was expecting a visitor—she accepted my nice, warm, comfy, fitting, clean, and elegant solution, but that was rare.

Her favorite color was navy, so one day I prepared something just the right color, and the right size.

"Yes, that's nice," Claire said, "but I keep wearing the same thing over and over again."

(I know that "over and over again" means "I want my favorite clothes.")

"Can't we put on these . . . these . . ." Clare looked for the word, for the series of sounds that represented a concept she clearly had in her head, and which I could guess:

"Trousers?"

"Yes!"

"Would you like these blue ones?" It was worth a try.

"No. Other ones . . ."

"Navy?" I was kind of hoping that by giving her a choice of colors, she might go for the ones that were good for her. But I wasn't in luck that day, because the answer was:

"No."

"Black?"

"Yes!"

Uh-oh, we're in trouble.

I knew the black trousers she meant. They were her favorite. It wasn't about the color, nor about the label. It was about the familiarity. She may have been losing her sight, and her memory of many things, but she knew her wardrobe well. And dementia wouldn't change that.

"Yes," Clare said. "Where are they?"

"They're right here, but they're too small. If you look at their size, it says ten, whereas you're wearing size fourteen now. The black trousers are smaller than your current body size. Does that make sense?"

"Let me try them."

"I am concerned you may find it disappointing, and I would rather save your time. Here are a pair of trousers in your current size, and here are the black ones, to compare. May I check whether the discrepancy between these sizes is visible to you?"

"Yes, the other ones are far too big for me. Let me try the black ones."

(Several minutes later she still couldn't put them on.)

"Let's try the blue ones," I said.

"They are too . . . too . . . big." (Her heavy, tragic *sigh*.)

Clare thought something was wrong with the trousers, something wrong with the washing machine, something wrong with whoever washed the trousers. The last time she remembered wearing them (which was about two years earlier), they had fit fine, and then very suddenly—literally overnight, from her point of view—they shrank. She didn't remember that we had tried them four times that week already, and that they did not fit. It was rare for Clare's dementia condition to allow her to reflect and wonder whether there may have been something wrong with her own perception, understanding, or memory. And of course, why would there be anything wrong with her mind? She had been able to make correct judgments all her adult life. Why should this be any different?

Anyway, I was being a good caregiver, I was exercising my patience, until I heard this:

"Why can't I wear my favorite black trousers? You haven't explained to me what on earth has happened to them?!"

Okay, my turn. This time, I sighed heavily in resignation. I felt as if my brain was frying. I felt tense. I heard criticism: I heard Clare accusing me of being the reason the trousers were no longer any good to her. My breath got shallower, my pulse quicker. We were nowhere near the end of this. Meanwhile, worry ran through my head that Clare was getting cold, as she had been sitting in her underwear for a considerable length of time now.

What's worse, my heart was getting cold too.

I was torn between respecting Clare's independence to choose what she wanted to wear, and caring for her well-being (regarding her body temperature). And for my own well-being, for that matter too.

I was getting desperate; I found it extremely hard to remain patient. Especially because it was a recurring scene. The repetition of the same conflict, over and over again, wore me down like sandpaper, little by little. I understood that people with dementia often don't learn from their mistakes, but I couldn't help thinking: Why can't she learn? Why can't she move on? I wish she could stop making the same mistake of yearning for clothes that don't fit her anymore. One day it's the black trousers, another day it's the flowery dress that she cannot put over her head anymore. I longed, at the least, for freshness, for some change to this pattern we got stuck in every tiresome morning.

Then I woke myself up internally: Hold on! Stop! Am I not making the same mistake over and over again myself? By getting annoyed, over and over again? Funny enough, every time she went after clothes that were undersized, I got triggered in the same way.

This was seriously boring.

While Clare scrutinized her unsuitable clothes again, I connected to my wish for both of us to be at ease. My approach, or strategy, of allowing myself to be driven by Clare's confusion while trying to help her meet her need for independence wasn't working—for me, or her for that matter. We were becoming disconnected. How could I tell? Because of my thoughts: If only you knew how much I have to put up with you! And her judgment: You are so unhelpful. You've done something to my favorite pair of trousers, and now they don't fit me. Why don't you admit it?

They were all fruitless accusations that were not getting us anywhere.

So I stopped, and acknowledged where I stood on the matter. "Clare . . . I am finding it very difficult," I said, in a tone of voice quite different from my "I'm the queen of patience" approach. This was the first time I had lost my patience, and also the first time I dared to express myself. And Clare looked at me attentively, trying to find out what this was all about. By expressing myself like this, showing myself to be vulnerable, I had broken a pattern between us. We were in new territory now.

"I am finding it difficult," I said, "because I think we've been in this room for about forty-five minutes now, and I am frustrated, because I so much wish for ease. I am also a bit worried that you may be getting cold." I was expressing emotion, and desperation, and above all the sadness in me that we kept finding ourselves in this same situation.

This is precisely what Clare picked up on. She heard me. It took her some minutes to process what I had said. I suspect it was unusual for her to hear someone express themselves as directly as I had. She was taken by surprise, and my experience told me this was always an advantage. Surprise opens something up—we have to stop and listen when something is said that is out of the ordinary. Since it is a surprise, we cannot predict what will happen next. And by changing the pattern, introducing surprise and uncertainty, I was meeting one of my needs: the need for freshness, and breaking the repetitive cycle.

But while we were certainly outside of the old pattern, we were not connected yet. I did not know where Clare was going. I didn't know what she heard me say, until she said this:

"It is hard for both of us, I know." And she reached out with her arm to stroke my back (which she missed, but never mind).

Her movement was clumsy, but her intention was pure. I felt like pure compassion was being poured onto me. "Do not worry, we will manage," she said, and we hugged, embracing ourselves and each other in mutual empathy.

Will I ever know how much Clare understood regarding those trousers? Might she have had any glimpse of recognition that these morning struggles had happened so very often? I think I will never know what prompted her compassionate response, other than the inherent goodness in her heart.

But you might be interested to hear what happened the next morning, and the morning after that. Well, Clare still wanted to put her too-small trousers on. She still noticed every tiny spot or fault in her blouses. But she stopped blaming me. She seemed to know I was a friend, to remember the feeling of being connected to me— even as we went on to play our dressing-room performances all over again. But we were so much more relaxed, the both of us. It was a bit like playing a game and getting carried away by it—but we always returned to a shared understanding that we were just playing.

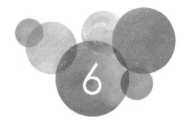

Feeding Inner Power

To the degree that we engage moment by moment in
the playfulness of enriching life . . . to that degree
we are being compassionate with ourselves.

—MARSHALL B. ROSENBERG, *American peacemaker*

A fundamental fact about the nature of every living thing is that they all need nurturing.

Humans, animals, and plants all require feeding. Each has a different preference as to what nurtures them, but the principle is the same. It is so basic that it is even shared with non-living things, like cars. A car's preference is fuel of some kind.

I used to be less keen on comparing people to machines. But I have realized that it is humans who make all these myriad different analogue or digital machines in our own image. They work like we do. It's not that we are like machines but rather that machines are like us.

After this realization, I began to see the study of mechanics of various modern inventions as ultimately a study of the human mind and heart. You can see some parallels between what is known as the mind-body problem in the way the software of a computer relates to its hardware. One is thought of as an operating system, running on its physical components. And as you will know if you have ever used a computer, a smartphone, or even a car, they all require care to keep running: charging, fueling, servicing. Power of some kind is required to get things going, whether it is a machine or an ungraspable human spirit.

As a caregiver I learned something about feeding my inner power through the analogy with a car. There are two ways to charge an electric car. One is to take it to an appropriate charging station and leave it alone for a while. Similarly, we caregivers can charge our inner power through self-empathy.

But there is another way forward: the car can charge itself while on the move. It can generate its own power through interaction.

You are not a car. But you have an inner power which is a renewable source of life force. It can be fed and it can grow, but first it must be acknowledged and taken care of.

FINDING POWER IN YOUR NEEDS

"I don't have my own needs," I hear some caregivers say. "I've sacrificed what I needed for what the person with dementia requires."

Some caregivers spend twenty-four hours a day with the person they look after. Others have that person on their mind at all times. Either way, a caregiver's mind is often filled with the person they care for. And this amount of time spent together can often create an illusion of "togetherness." We substitute frequency of contact for connection. I can easily convince myself that I am connected with someone merely because they rely on me so much and we are in such frequent contact. But unless my heart is in it, all we've got between us is dependency.

Paradoxically, in order to truly connect with another person, I must first become a person in my own right. This does not mean abandoning the person I care about—it doesn't even mean being separate from them. It means acknowledging that my own needs are distinct from what my relationship with that person requires. That's the only way I know of truly enriching a dementia relationship. Because when I assume that connection means merging with another to the extent that I forget my own distinctness, I impoverish my relationship as well as myself.

I may think that I know what the other person needs, and what's good for them. When I was stuck with Clare in her dressing room, I often worried that she was getting cold. So I thought it was good for her to get dressed as quickly as possible. But was it? Had she ever said she felt bothered by the cold? I may have thought I knew her needs and what was good for her, and was convinced that I was acting in Clare's best interest by trying to speed things up. But wasn't I perhaps trying to meet my own need for efficiency, instead? I thought that if only she could get dressed quickly, she would be happy and everything would be okay. Somehow I hoped we might be more connected if only she did what I thought was best for her.

In a survey of clients of the care agency I worked for, people regularly reported how uneasy they felt around their caregivers. "She is wonderful, don't get me wrong, very caring and dedicated, but God, she can talk! Chatting all day long, as if she's trying to keep me cheerful at all times." For the cared for, the ability to disconnect may be their last resort: disconnecting from the person trying to make them happy at all costs is one way they can declare their independence and autonomy.

And I know caregivers who assume that people with dementia are depressed or lonely and therefore require constant company, entertainment, and chit-chat. In some cases, it may even be true. The question I needed to ask myself as a caregiver was this: Whose need am I trying to meet, the other person's or my own?

Caregiving is not everyone's first choice for a walk of life. It is often more a necessity than a calling. It might seem that given a choice, most caregivers would do something different with their lives. Or would they?

Ask yourself why you provide care for someone. If you find yourself saying that you have to, then keep asking. Why? Why do you have to? Do you do it because of love? Out of respect or affection? Is it because you care? Or is it a way to contribute to your family? Whatever your answer is, it will be either a need you have yourself, or a strategy to fulfill one of your needs.

For me, taking up duty as a live-in caregiver and companion was a way to support myself and my academic studies financially— at first. But the reason I stayed on for five years was because doing so fulfilled many of my own values and principles. I enjoyed being trustworthy and competent. I met my needs for empowerment and recognition by putting myself in situations where others could rely on me and in which I could be helpful to them. Caregiving in itself can indeed be a way to enrich your own life, not only that of the person you care for.

But caregiving did not meet all of my needs all at once. There were times when I felt downhearted and helpless, and sometimes even scared and vulnerable. And it wasn't until I admitted to myself that I had other needs—such as choice, equality, and ease—that I was able to find other ways of fulfilling those needs, outside of the caregiving role. And that was empowering my dementia relationship, though indirectly.

Knowing what it was that I needed fed my inner power. Yes, taking responsibility for your own feelings and needs requires some courage. Taking responsibility without blaming someone or something isn't for the fainthearted. It requires clarity to recognize that others are not responsible for making you feel better.

I spent time telling myself that Clare was a bit stubborn and uncooperative in her dressing room. The more I believed my story, the slower she became, and the less my need for efficiency was met. Instead I could have taken a more straightforward approach. I could have followed the signpost of my irritation, owned that feeling, and acknowledged that being efficient mattered to me. It was my need, not Clare's stubbornness, that was popping up in the form of irritation. But it was scary to admit to myself that I was irritated because I feared being blamed for not being efficient *and* as patient and forbearing as I thought a good caregiver should be. The very first step in accepting my feelings and needs was admitting to myself that I was a little scared to own the feelings and needs that were alive for me.

Caregiving requires a brave heart. Nonviolent Communication, as a discipline of the heart, is a process—not a technique, not a method, but a process—that can help. Because in Nonviolent Communication, we take responsibility for our own well-being. And we do that by keeping an awareness of our needs and trusting in our heart. In other words, we build our ability to see clearly, feel our feelings, sense our needs, and request strategies to meet those needs.

Commitment to clear Observation, felt Feeling, sensed Need, and fulfilling Strategy constitutes the Nonviolent Communication process.

As time goes on and dementia develops, someone with dementia gradually becomes inseparable from their caregiver, yet both remain distinct individuals. When I acknowledge my needs as my own, I am in a much better position to connect with the other person.

The following stories are examples of how awareness of my own needs benefited both me and my client, and consequently enriched our relationship. Although each time I started off assuming that I was doing something for the other person, admitting that I was trying to meet my own needs was eventually both sobering and wholesome. Once I realized this—usually after a little prompt from my client—I was able to find a strategy that worked for me, and that turned my own needs into a gift to our dementia relationship.

Ultimately it is lack of awareness of our own needs that gets us into trouble. Because when we know and own our needs, we can find peaceful ways of fulfilling them.

TUNING YOUR STRATEGIES

Spending day after day mostly indoors at Yvonne's house, which she had such a love-hate relationship with, I found myself weary and bored at times. And I thought that Yvonne could also do with a bit of a change. Her best friend, Gabi, agreed that it would be nice for all of us to have some fun together. Gabi and I were on the same page, "Fun is important for everyone, and Yvonne really needs a breath of fresh air and some enjoyment." We settled on going for a drive, and Yvonne went along with the idea.

As I described to her how excited I felt about the three of us going out, it seemed to me at first that she really connected with the joy she could read on my face. But in hindsight, I don't think she really comprehended the idea of going for a drive as a way to have fun. "Fun" sounds good in theory, but so much depends on how each individual's need for fun is met.

We took Yvonne in the car, along with a wheelchair in the trunk and excitement on our faces, and went for a ride around the neighborhood where she had spent most of her life. The day was lovely, the sunny day so encouraging, and Gabi and I full of such uplifted spirits.

It didn't take long for us to realize that for Yvonne, this supposedly fun activity felt like her own personal *Back to the Future 2* movie—in which she was transported out of her own time to drive through a world thirty years in the future. As far as she was concerned, the present time was around 1960, and she was witnessing a futuristic film set. Was this some kind of joke? And unlike the actual *Back to the Future 2* movie, it wasn't a comedy—far from it. Yvonne was not amused at seeing houses built all over the rolling hills she used to go for walks on. The whole area was densely inhabited, and everyone seemed to have a car! And that was wrong, according to Yvonne. Everything was wrong. For Yvonne, the world fifty years earlier was her world, whereas our contemporary world was an unreal vision of horror—unfamiliar, foreign, unpleasant, and crowded. Not her idea of fun at all.

Since that memorable trip, Gabi and I have learned that when we do things that aim to meet our needs, we have to try to imagine what that will be like for Yvonne. We need to stretch our imagination far enough to imagine the world from a 1960s perspective. If I have a need for fun, I have to own that need, and claim it as important for me. And if I want to contribute to Yvonne's sense of fun, it has to be on her terms. I cannot make her happy by aiming to meet my own need through my own strategy. It's like me drinking water and expecting to quench Yvonne's thirst. Even though we all, as human beings, have a need for fun, change, or enjoyment, a particular need may be alive for ourselves but not necessarily for everyone else.

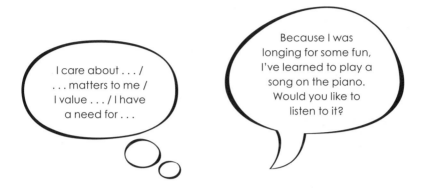

After realizing that it was important for me to have some fun, I also wanted to contribute to Yvonne's well-being and uplifted spirit. I knew she loved piano music, and I wanted to learn the piano myself. She already had a piano at her house, so I was all set for the adventure of learning how to play the thing. I started by practicing every day, for eight days, following instructions from a YouTube channel.

Not exactly a musical education that would take me to the greatest concert halls in the world, I know. But learning was so much fun, it was a reward in itself for my hard work (a whole weeks' worth!). And one day, when I felt ready, I invited Yvonne and Gabi to my performance.

I may have been ready, but the world certainly wasn't. I believe it took a good dose of openness for Gabi to sit with a straight face and witness my impersonation of a pianist. I could almost hear her thinking, Have mercy on my aging ears! But Yvonne was spellbound, tapping her finger as if she were imitating a metronome, which kept the rhythm for me. (What rhythm? Gabi might have asked.) Then there was clapping, and laughing faces— some laughing with others, some laughing at others. The point is, all of us were laughing.

Yvonne did not seem to remember anything about the piano performance later that day, and yet she was in good spirits. She had no memory, but I believe the feeling of rejuvenation remained. With dementia, feelings are more faithful to reality, while memories distort and misrepresent it. Yvonne's reality was bright that evening, though there was one thing that seemed to worry her: "You must remind me to call someone to look at my piano. I think it is horribly out of tune!"

With dementia, feelings are more faithful to reality, while memories distort and misrepresent it.

RECOGNIZING YOUR OWN NEEDS

Trying to disguise your strategy of meeting your own need as supposedly addressing another person's needs doesn't pay off. No matter how many abilities your friend with dementia has lost, they can tell the difference between their interests and yours.

Dory started wearing hearing aids, after a long period of not recognizing that her hearing had dramatically decreased. She remembered that she had hearing aids—well, sometimes. When she did remember, she was protective about them. She cared very much about not losing them, apart from the fairly frequent occasions when she forgot she had them on (while getting into the shower) or where she had put them. To my knowledge she had two pairs of hearing aids that got lost, or damaged in some way. As a result, her long-term friend and live-in caregiver asked her to take the hearing aids out before she went to bed.

While her friend was away on vacation, I came to stay with Dory for a few weeks. I was instructed to look after the hearing aids overnight, as that was when the previous pair had gone missing.

"May I have your hearing aids, Dory?" I asked.

"Why? What would you need them for?"

"I would like to take care of them for you."

"No, no need. I will take them out when I'm ready to sleep. And I am not ready yet."

"Would you like me to come back when you are ready?"

"No, I will be okay."

"You know, if I took them now, I could give them a good cleaning for you. They should be cleaned on a daily basis, and I would like to help."

"I know. I can do it. I'm okay."

"I am a little concerned," I said, "that they may accidentally go missing. You may, for example, fall asleep, not realizing you left them in."

"Are you suggesting I am not capable of looking after myself? I have never lost hearing aids, and I have had them for years. I don't need your assistance. You can relax and go to bed."

Well, now it was time for me to stop pretending that I wanted to take the hearing aids to help Dory. I was trying to meet my own need here: my need for ease and comfort. Taking the hearing aids would save me the worry that Dory might put them somewhere so "safe" that neither of us would be able to find them again. It wasn't in my interest for Dory to lose them again. I would have to shout every time we had a conversation for her to be able to hear me at all.

I was also aware that she would probably be upset if they went missing again—but only if she remembered having them to begin with. So at the end of the day, I needed to admit that I was requesting the hearing aids from Dory to meet my need for ease, and stop pretending my request was an offer to help her out.

I also knew that as soon as I admitted my need, and that my request was to contribute to my own peace of mind, she had the right to say no. This could not be a demand: I would not manipulate Dory into something she wasn't ready to do.

The discipline of Nonviolent Communication is not intended to be used to make someone do something you want them to do. For two reasons: First, no matter how much we fantasize about making people do things, like wash the dishes, we wouldn't want the same to be done to us. Would we want to be made to do things? Manipulated by some communication technique? Second, and more important, if it were truly possible to manipulate someone, our relationship with that person would not be more alive, it would be more automatic. Not really a living relationship, but a series of knee-jerk reactions.

So, Dory was a free person and might not be interested in meeting my need for ease by giving me her hearing aids. And that was an option too.

I went to the kitchen to get Dory some fresh water, and when I came back, she was getting ready for bed. I addressed her again, and this time I said what I meant, and meant what I said:

"Dory, you know your hearing aids . . . "

"What about them?"

At this point I wondered if she had already forgotten our conversation fifteen minutes earlier.

"Because it would meet my need for ease, would you be willing to give them to me to look after overnight?"

"Sure, if it will make you feel more at ease. You can take them. But where did I put them? Did you take them out already?"

"No, I think you still have them in your ears."

"Oh, yes. That's right. Here they are, you can have them. I hope it will give you peace of mind."

It did indeed. But peace of mind wasn't the only thing we gained that night. We built trust, connected through our expressed needs, acknowledged our freedom to say no, and strengthened our relationship. This isn't always easy—but it's mostly easier than you might expect. Expressing your needs openly is an option. At times you may find that doing so benefits both you and the person you care for. In this way, your distinct personal needs and values can feed your inner power, which enhances your dementia relationship. For better, and for worse.

Savoring Hurt, Guilt, and Grief

Where your pain is, there your heart lies also.

—ANNA KAMIEŃSKA, *Polish poet*

Where there is a way to think positively about dementia, so there is also a way to think negatively about it, and there may even seem to be more evidence to support a negative outlook than a positive one.

To fight pessimism, many people try to keep a positive attitude toward dementia, and keep the gloominess at bay, at all costs and at all times. Liv Larsson, a Swedish author and certified trainer with the Center for Nonviolent Communication, says that positive thinking is often used to try to escape the pain and grief that exists in our lives. On the other hand, I find that negativity turns the natural pain of life into a torture of suffering, making things worse than they are. Larsson finds that both positive and negative thinking present distorted views. Making everything out to be exclusively black or white limits the full color of life.

An honest approach to dementia, I believe, is to savor its

bittersweet flavor. In this approach we accept the full spectrum of tastes, without denying its bitterness nor exaggerating its sweetness. It takes courage to taste life as it comes. Barbara Ehrenreich says in her book *Bright-Sided: How the Relentless Promotion of Positive Thinking Has Undermined America*, "There is a vast difference between positive thinking and existential courage."

Beyond doubt, life with dementia comes with a degree of bitterness. Caregiving often takes place amid distress and helplessness but the difficult experiences of hurt, guilt, and grief don't have to spoil your dementia relationship. They inevitably are already part of it.

As you develop an ability to savor all the flavors of life, you may be surprised to find some sweetness to be enjoyed *in* the poignancy of painful experiences. Without trying to sugarcoat that which is difficult to swallow or digest, you can simply be honest.

Honesty is primarily an attitude of inclusivity, of accepting and acknowledging what's there. It's about being real, and true to who you are, and how you are—true, most importantly, to yourself. This transparent openness to yourself, along with the warmth of self-empathy, creates the conditions for the sweetness of connection to occur. And as you may have already experienced, hard episodes in life, when shared, can become a binding factor in a relationship.

> *Honesty is primarily an attitude of inclusivity, of accepting and acknowledging what's there.*

In a dementia relationship, you will very likely face judgmental accusations, feelings of blame and failure, and denial of responsibility. Unfortunately, we can't expect someone with dementia to watch their own tongue and improve their own attitude. Their ability to engage in this type of reflection is probably limited by their illness. So I find it is usually up to me, as a caregiver, to take a step back and look at the situation from a bigger perspective. As we explored in Part One of this book, it is possible to focus both our attention and imagination on wholeness, and to choose wholesome responses to what life with dementia throws at us. The way we savor our feelings of hurt, guilt, and grief can enrich the flavor of the relationship for both parties. Thus, in taking care of yourself, you take care of the person you care about too.

We wouldn't feel hurt and sorrow if we didn't care in the first place. This vulnerability is at the heart of authentic caregiving, and at the same time, it is the quality which enables connection to be honest and real. Daniel J. Siegel has said that to care for people is to care about them. And so it happens that when you care about someone with dementia, sorrow and grief will be part of your relationship to a greater or lesser degree. Your dementia relationship can take these bitter ingredients and contain them. The stronger your relationship, the sweeter the aftertaste that remains.

HEARING BEYOND YOUR HURT

"Don't focus on what other people think of you. Believe me, you'll live longer," Marshall B. Rosenberg liked to say. I had occasion to remember these words one day with Yvonne. I discovered that I could choose where to focus my attention—on her words, or on her heart. The more I was able to pay attention to what was alive in her heart, the bigger my heart could grow—big enough to contain both myself and her in it. It was no longer single-sized, it had grown to be suitable for two.

Yvonne appeared fragile and frail to those who did not know her. But what they didn't see at first glimpse was the strength of her character. She could scream at the top of her voice. "You wretched, stupid people," she yelled that day. "You keep me in here against my will. I will call the police!" And she did.

I was in the other room when I heard her say to the police officer on the other end of the line, "These people, they are wicked, bad people. Criminals! They are tyrants, keeping me captive in this awful, awful house!"

Hearing this left me in quite an aggrieved mental state. For all the effort I'd put into trying to meet her needs, to comfort her! And even though I knew she confused some past experiences with the present, I still was shocked and disappointed to hear her describing me with adjectives such as *wretched*, *stupid*, and *bad*.

Why would she say such things? I asked myself. Why is she doing this to me?

Then there were the worries: What if the police believed her? She was, after all, frail and defenseless, and therefore must be assumed to be innocent. And therefore I must be the villain. What if they came and arrested me as a suspect in a kidnapping? What would everyone think?

And what about my reputation?! If I really was such a good caregiver as people thought, surely she wouldn't be saying all these horrible things to the officials. They would have to write up a report that mentions my name.

The torture of asking "why" and "what if" was a signal that woke me up. It reminded me to connect empathically with myself. For my own sake, and for my own comfort, I stopped listening to Yvonne's phone conversation, and directed my attention within myself. There I sensed my tension and unease.

Instead of suppressing my feelings, I made enough room for them within me. I acknowledged how upset, resentful, and worried I was. These feelings, once I listened, informed me of my underlying needs. I was longing for trust and recognition, and to be seen and appreciated.

I wanted to be acknowledged and trusted because appreciation and trust are qualities within me. Once I realized that, I could connect with those qualities right away. Like a moon which is whole, whether visible in its entirety or not. When I shed some light on my inherent qualities, I began to feel relief from my distress, and felt whole again.

From this perspective things started looking and sounding different. Even Yvonne sounded different. At first I was confused why she kept referring to "these" people, her "wretched" caregivers? I was the only other person in the house. Was she referring to her previous helpers, or did I multiply in her mind?

But then I realized she wasn't speaking about me at all. She was expressing her feelings.

When she said, "These wretched people, they don't care about me. All they care about is getting my money!" I no longer heard hurtful accusations. I heard her expressing something else: I'm scared. Am I safe? Can I trust the people who look after me? And when she said, "I want them to go away!" this is what I heard: I'm longing to be independent again. I wish I could decide for myself.

Focusing on Yvonne's needs, not on the words she spoke, made it possible for me to see her actions in a new light. Indeed, after allowing myself a few minutes for self-empathy, my imagination snapped back in focus.

From then on—but not before!—I was able to listen empathically to what was going on for Yvonne. I guessed that after she dozed off that afternoon, she woke up not recognizing her house again. She may have felt frightened, and she may have felt that she needed help and support. She had learned in her life that when something frightening happens, when you believe you are endangered, you call 911. So I can only imagine how much she was longing for support and reassurance! At the same time, perhaps there was a bit of desire to be in full command of her life and how she spent her days, to be self-sufficient again and autonomous.

It made a lot of sense to me, and the more I was able to imagine Yvonne's perspective, the more connected I felt to her. Even before I went back to her room, while I was still waiting outside her door, I felt better. Mysteriously, being able to hear Yvonne empathically recharged my own batteries.

By the time I heard her finishing the conversation and putting the phone down, I was able to come into her room calmly, though still not knowing what to expect!

"Oh, there you are! I was so terrified!" Yvonne said. "Where were you?"

I came closer and held her hand. "It's all right now," I said. "I hear you've been stressed and needed support. I am here." And Yvonne clung to my hand, with an expression of gratitude painted all over her face.

That was such a relief—for both of us, I think. But after all the complaints I'd heard directed at me, this moment was possible only because I had been listening for what was alive: first in me, and then in her. Because I was able, even with some difficulty, to hear empathically.

In case you were wondering, the police never came. Later I learned from Yvonne's family that the police had her number on record: it wasn't the first time they'd received a call like that from her. But I believe Yvonne and I were both very glad for each other's company that evening.

OUTGROWING YOUR GUILT

Guilt is a funny sort of feeling. On one hand, it so often relates to chocolate, or television comedies. On the other hand, it does not make us laugh. It makes us feel miserable and tense. And yet, one of the top three responses in Google Search to what we feel most guilty about is . . . relaxation. Even though we know we need time off to rest and relax, guilt seems to be programmed into our system. Especially if we try to use leisure to escape from the blaming thoughts that haunt us.

Fran is a practitioner of Nonviolent Communication who shared with me her feelings of guilt around her friend, Diamantina, who was living in a nursing home. Diamantina had been an influential figure in Fran's years of adolescence. "She was there for me when my own parents didn't know how to support me in the challenges I was facing back then. Now it should be my time to be there for her," Fran said.

We may feel guilty about a friend, a mother or father, or anyone else. We might be thinking: I know I am not spending enough time with her. Or: When they were looking after me, they were so much more patient. Or: He's my closest family, it shouldn't be strangers that take care of him when he needs me most. Trying to relax while keeping all this self-blame at bay takes an awful lot of energy. It's a vicious circle of guilt which plays on our mind, like a background app using up battery life. No wonder we can't quite let go and put our feet up. And at the end of this energetically draining activity, we haven't become any more useful to the people we care for!

Guilt gets in the way of authenticity. It derails connection into guilt trips.

Sure, we often use guilt to make ourselves put more effort into relating to someone with dementia, or to go and visit them more often. But is it ever enough? Do we ever live up to the expectations our judgmental minds demand? Are we truly able to be present with the person we care for while we are consumed by guilt? And, tragically, how often does this whole performance of "doing the right thing" leave us exhausted and avoiding the person we're feeling guilty about?

Avoidance often happens whenever we are motivated by guilt. We may try to put on a cheerful face to mask our own suffering, but dementia challenges us to stop being nice and start being real with others and ourselves. And guilt gets in the way of this authenticity. It derails attempts at connection into guilt trips. Connection dwells in the present. If we get distracted by guilty worries about the past or the future, we will be disconnected from what matters right in front of us.

Fran finally got in touch with her feelings. She felt how much Diamantina meant to her, and how hard it had been for Fran to carry on with her own life, traveling abroad and leaving her friend behind. "It touches me deeply, but it is okay. I am comfortable with this pain," Fran said, as tears ran down her cheeks. She was saturated with feelings of grief, sadness, gratitude, and tenderness, all of which had been buried under the heavy weight of guilt. Had Fran allowed the grief to weigh her down, she would have become depressed. Instead, her feelings sprouted and rose above the burden of guilt, and she used it as soil from which to flourish into the wealth of things that mattered to both Fran and Diamantina. "She was a strong, independent women who often told me that she felt she had had a wonderful life." As Fran reflected on their friendship, she realized they both valued independence, vitality, and adventure. She learned to trust their connection and the needs they had in common. "I know she would have told me, 'Fran, go and make the most of your life.' It almost feels like this is what she's trying to tell me when I meet her nowadays too."

Regular visits to Diamantina are still part of Fran's life, yet whenever she travels away, she remains connected to her dear friend, no matter how far she goes. To paraphrase William James, we are like islands in the sea, who appear separate on the surface, but are connected in the deep.

Trusting in connection allows us to deeply care about someone and to look after our own needs—for relaxation, or for adventure. We cannot bypass the natural pain of life—the pain of change and transformation. Such pain is natural in the way giving birth, growing teeth, or having a period is painful. This pain does not indicate that there is something wrong with you or your relationships. It comes with life, naturally. Often it indicates growth. But it is up to you whether you allow the guilt to bury you alive, or whether you grow out of it.

Once you allow yourself to experience the pain of life, to feel the burden of guilt, sorrow, and regret, you can use it as soil. The dark place you find yourself in can easily be misinterpreted as a grave. But consider that perhaps you have been planted. All seeds start growing in darkness before sprouting into the light. Being well rooted in the reality of pain, we can rise above it, for much more satisfying and deep connections with ourselves and with others. We can then become genuinely interested in the world beyond our own struggles.

FEELING YOUR GRIEF

Dementia can be experienced as loss. Loss of abilities and skills. Loss of a relationship that you used to have. You may have had a parent-child relationship where roles were defined, and now it is not at all clear who is playing which role. Similarly, between every two people, whether lovers, siblings, or friends, there is a dynamic in which each person has a role to play. In the play of dementia, the script has gone missing, or got terribly muddled. People say, "My father has become my child" or "I am mothering my older sister" or "My husband is now my patient." These are ways people describe how their roles have changed and how they are redefining the character of their relationship. It's a new relationship now—which can become a wholesome dementia relationship. But it's hard to appreciate it fully until we allow ourselves to experience the loss and grieve the past. We need to do this in order to meet the present.

We acknowledge our needs either through celebrating or through mourning.

As it happens, loss is precisely one of the ways in which we experience our needs. Sometimes we experience our needs as fulfilled, and we can celebrate them. At other times we experience needs as unfulfilled, and we can mourn them. In either case, we acknowledge our needs, whether through celebrating or through mourning.

There are many needs I may be fulfilling in my caregiving role, and perhaps just as many which I hold unfulfilled. Acknowledging our unfulfilled needs, unsatisfied longings, and unmet values is part of the Nonviolent Communication process which rests on the principle of honest inclusivity.

Grief is a type of self-empathy. Its purpose is to reconnect us to the aliveness within us, even if in the context of death. It is never too late to grieve, even if the relationship you grieve or the person you miss died decades ago. Grief can be postponed, but it cannot be canceled. You can resurrect the connection and fulfill your needs by addressing what's alive in you now. If there is still some pain, or sadness, or even resignation, that's your magic spark. In addressing the past we always look for what's alive—here and now—and pay empathic attention to our present feelings and needs. Because grief is not the business of the past, nor of the future. No matter how old the pain, the healing of it is fresh and brings us back to life. And the healed pain of disconnection is accompanied by a deep relief and acceptance.

In this very moment, as I remember my long-gone Grandma Maria, I feel regret and a kind of sorrow that I wasn't able to approach her then in the way I have learned since to approach people with dementia. I wish I'd had the skills back then to build a solid dementia relationship with my own relative. When I feel sadness fill my heart, I realize how much it matters to me to contribute to the lives of others meaningfully. This is my need for contribution.

I recognize this need by noticing how I feel while I'm wishing to change the past. But it is not a past need—it is alive and present. It is an aspiration for my present life.

I can wake up to my needs by accepting my sadness in the present moment. My friend Ian Mackenzie campaigns for recognition of the value of sadness. He says that running around looking for happiness is mostly running away from sadness— and therefore, running away from life, of which sadness is an inescapable part.

There's plenty to feel sad about, plenty of loss in dementia. Having a loved one whose dementia drastically changed the nature of your relationship may feel confusing. Even though the person, your relative or friend, is still in their body, you may struggle to find "the real them" inside. They don't act the same way. Often it isn't only behavior that's changed but also their personality. You may find yourself saying, The person I once knew is gone, or He isn't himself anymore, or She may as well be dead, or The body is there, but nothing more. Although the subject of these expressions appears to be about them—the person with dementia—your thoughts are still more about you than about them. This is the way you're expressing your underlying feelings, your way of grieving.

Bereavement comes in various shades. It's your grief: feel it your way.

You may feel dejected, heartbroken, or filled with melancholy. Or you may be furious, helpless, and angry. Bereavement comes in various shades, and at different temperatures ranging from cold resignation to hot indignation. It's your grief: feel it your way.

Grief will take you to the fine line between rawness and enjoyment—a state of vulnerability. But if you try to *think* rather than *feel* your grief, it will only increase your suffering; it won't address the pain you're experiencing. Thoughts might sound like this: Why did it happen to her? It's not fair! Or: I have to get over this quicker. I have to get on with my life.

Whenever we complain, grasp our loss intellectually, or mourn in the "right" way, we are not present to what is alive in us. Over-thinking is a sort of distraction, which instead of bringing relief, causes suffering. Whereas grief is not about proliferating suffering, but about getting in touch with our pain. There are no words that will take the pain away.

If there is a feeling that is neither happy nor sad, a feeling right in between pleasant and unpleasant, that would be poignancy. Feeling poignant is what I experience when I mourn wholesomely. In those moments I am, as a result of the grieving process, neither depressed about life nor jumping with joy. In poignancy we embrace life with its sorrows and all its painful, challenging, intriguing beauty. It's an experience of stillness.

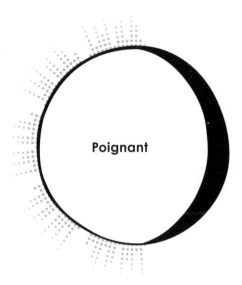

Kathleen Macferran, a certified trainer with the Center for Nonviolent Communication, experienced a double loss as both of her parents had dementia. She had grown up with a continuous sense that her parents had her back, that they provided her with a safety net she could always fall back into. Then things changed, and Kathleen realized it was her turn to provide support. The roles got shuffled; responsibilities were divided in a new way. In adapting to all the changes and role swaps, Kathleen also became aware of grief around her ancestral roots.

Her parents were losing memories—memories about the family, stories about the past, and tales of ancestors. They lost not only their own memories but the memories that Kathleen felt were her heritage. Pieces of her past were missing. The collective family memory was substantially impoverished. One whole generation's remembrance, represented by her father and mother's collection of memories, was wiped out. In mourning this loss, Kathleen connected with her own deep sadness, and the unfulfilled quality of belonging.

In her grieving process, she also recognized the loneliness

she was experiencing in relation to her father. Memories of his keen interest in the things Kathleen was passionate about, and the lively conversations and discussions they used to have, now had an aftertaste of bereavement. With his progressing illness, he became less outgoing; he no longer reached out to her with questions expressing his interest in her activities. The value of sharing and mutuality was another that Kathleen mourned lovingly.

When we lose a relationship in its earlier form, we lose the types of activities and conversations we used to enjoy. We lose a whole lifestyle we used to think of as so integral to who we are and how we want to be in the world. We lose an imagined future together. We say goodbye to our past together as someone lets go of one memory after another. All this makes us think the person we used to know is gone. But it is our former relationship that is gone. We are grieving the relationship that we used to have.

As for the person who has dementia, yes, they've changed. But it isn't that they no longer are *who* they used to be as much as that they aren't *how* they used to be. They are new, and so are you. Your relationship, your new relationship, needs you both—not the old ones, but *the way you are now.* Your dementia relationship is the updated version of your former relationship.

Undoubtedly in most cases, it is immensely sad. There may be so much sadness and grief that it takes longer than you, or anyone around you, wants to schedule for it. Grief takes time, and it takes sensitivity. It may be equally painful to watch as it is to feel. Lama Shenpen Hookham, a Buddhist teacher, has said that our approach to grief often reflects our approach to self-empathy. "It is insensitive to try to get the bereaved to 'move on' or 'let go' . . . When people do this, it is probably their own feelings of fear, inadequacy, and impatience talking. . . . If that person has been insensitive to themselves in bereavement, they are likely to be insensitive to others."

Another way to put it is that the sweetness of connection can be tasted first in our own difficult and painful experiences. It wasn't until I developed a taste for connection within myself that I felt myself truly able to connect with another person. Self-connection is an anchor for a satisfying dementia relationship, with all its possible ups and downs: it provides stability and centeredness for both people involved.

Once you've tasted the sweetness of connection for yourself, you will hunger for more. That's when you can learn how to receive more from the other person, in whatever way they choose to enrich your life.

PART THREE

LISTENING WITH HEART

Caregiving offers continual opportunities for creativity. With empathic imagination, you will learn to listen to more than words. Because connection doesn't require language. It can also be found through music, silence, presence, and touch.

HOW TO CONNECT WITH SOMEONE WHO HAS DEMENTIA

- Be curious about their world. What might it be like there?
- Practice wondering: What matters to this person at this moment?
- Acknowledge their illness to yourself, and acknowledge their feelings and needs to them.
- Find imaginative solutions to unmet needs that are expressed by distress, anger, or aggression.
- Recognize old repetition as an opportunity to try something new.
- Use questions that open a conversation further: What was that like? Was it fun? Was it scary? Will you tell me more?
- Allow time. Respect another person's rhythm.
- Seek connection both with and without words.

Being Curious

And those who were seen dancing were thought to be
insane by those who could not hear the music.

—FRIEDRICH NIETZSCHE, *German philosopher*

We take for granted the world as it appears to our senses. Sight, sound, smell, taste, feeling—the information our senses present is, by definition, the way we see the world. But these senses may deliver different information to someone with dementia. Those of us who don't have dementia need to use our imagination with intent, to understand how the world is experienced by those who do have dementia.

I mean this literally as well as figuratively. Literally, what would the world look like if you could not perceive depth, if you never knew whether the surface ahead was flat or had steps? Figuratively, what would it feel like to live with a condition that affected your ability to think, move, perceive, and understand the world around you?

I can't tell you what it is like, nor would any person with dementia be able to speak for everyone else living with the condition. Dementia is a very personal matter. The only person who will be able to tell you how they perceive the world, and what they care about, is the person who has dementia. Once you see them as experts on themselves and their own dementia, you may become even more interested in their experience.

People's behavior may be awkward at times, and they may demand the impossible or make irrational comments. But if you listen attentively, you will hear that they are telling you what makes their life worth living, their music worth dancing to. The word *ear* can be found in the word *(h)ear(t)*. You can listen with your heart—listen to the core of the other person, not only to their words. Tune in to what moves them and fills them with song.

WONDERING INTO ANOTHER'S WORLD

Teachers of Nonviolent Communication like myself often suggest that the best way to establish life-enriching, empathic communication with other people is to start with a neutral observation of reality. Observation is the very first commitment in Nonviolent Communication, followed by Feeling, Need, and Request. These four commitments compose the Nonviolent Communication process which we can use both to connect with oneself and to connect with others. To communicate with someone who is living with dementia, we need to add some empathic imagination to it.

Let's think about this for a minute. To make a neutral observation of any situation, you're most likely to use one of your senses. What is it that you saw? What do you remember yourself or another person doing or saying? What is it that you heard?

With most people in my life, I can communicate more clearly by starting with a neutral observation: I recall you saying that you would wash the dishes. Rather than a judgment or analysis:

As usual, you left all the work to me. But with someone who has dementia, my observation of even the simplest situation may not overlap with their experience at all.

An observation, you see, relies on memory, on the physical senses, and on the listener's agreement that these constitute objective reality. If I say that I saw unwashed dishes in the sink, I expect the listener to agree that at the time mentioned, there were indeed unwashed dishes in the sink. If I say that I remember hearing them say earlier that they would wash the dishes, I expect the listener to agree that's what they said, especially if they only have to remember as far back as earlier that evening.

In a dementia relationship, we cannot expect such observations to be neutral meeting places. A person with dementia may not recall what I recall, may not see, hear, or sense the same things I do. If so, this person is highly unlikely to anticipate the same outcomes I do. As a result, at any point, either party may find the other person's "neutral observation" highly triggering. The person I expected to wash the dishes may have started a load of laundry instead. They might be genuinely surprised when I inquire about their earlier promise of washing the dishes. What dishes? What sink? What are you talking about?

So instead of "neutral observation" in our dementia relationships, let's try "empathic imagination." Empathic imagination is focused on discovering what's real, not what's imaginary. It is not about reading other people's minds and ignorantly assuming we know what they think and feel. Empathic imagination means we have a genuine interest in what may be happening for another person, and we make a respectful attempt to understand

Empathic imagination is a respectful attempt to understand what someone may be experiencing.

what they may be experiencing, through their feelings and needs. It means being curious about their world.

People may have odd ways of going about things. They may put an electric kettle directly on the stovetop, or dirty dishes into the washing machine. But when we are curious enough, we may find that these seemingly absurd behaviors make sense in their world. If I try to imagine myself in the world of someone like Yvonne, who lives in the reality of the 1960s, when there were no electric kettles, her behavior might seem perfectly reasonable. Likewise, someone like Gordon might confuse the washing machine for a dishwasher.

When you learn to see things from their perspective, I think you'll find it much easier to connect.

"People here are as nutty as a fruitcake, you know," Sian confided to her son in a lowered voice, while making sure no one in the lounge overheard. But she could not hide the gesture of her finger swirling by her head. "You know, mad as a hatter!" she said, and her son smiled.

Sian is an Alzheimer's patient in a dementia nursing home in Wales, and as far as she is concerned, she is the only sane person in the nuthouse. Indeed, people diagnosed with mental illness such as dementia generally don't perceive themselves as crazy. No more than you and I see ourselves as mad.

When we become curious about the needs that people are trying to meet for themselves, we hear their sanity, their wholeness—regardless of their abilities or disabilities. The Chinese philosopher Chuang-Tzu said that true empathy requires listening with the whole being. Such empathy listens for what's whole in the other person—wholeheartedly. With this empathic skill we can form a wholesome relationship with anyone.

To make a delicious dementia relationship you will need the following ingredients: an appropriate touch, a pinch of imagination, and a big heart. (Don't worry, you can grow it bigger if you are worried your own heart may not be big enough. As long as you've got one, that's all you need.) Although a dementia relationship can be tough at times, with some empathy, it can crack your hearts open—your own heart and that of the person you care for. No matter how nutty you both seem.

Ingredients for a delicious dementia relationship: an appropriate touch, a pinch of imagination, and a big heart.

My friend Ruth's mother Jane has dementia and has been living in a residential home since she began to need care around the clock. She is otherwise fit and unaware of any difficulties with her mental abilities. She does not understand why she was moved into a nursing home and thinks it is perhaps because she had been a nuisance to her family. "I promise I won't be any trouble, just get me home," she says to Ruth. "I will keep out of everyone's way and live in the cellar."

Ruth has been developing a habit of self-empathy, which translated into her ability to listen with heart. It wasn't easy, but she was able at times to listen to her mother's heartbreaking plea calmly and carefully, without contradicting or interrupting her or trying to convince her that the nursing home was better for her. Ruth simply stayed curious about what her mother was longing for. In other words, she listened for the needs underlying what her mother was saying.

This is hard to do. But no matter how pointless certain words or behaviors may seem to us, they are always aiming at something significant enough to be worth pursuing. Being curious requires natural stillness, rather than jumping to conclusions, and assumptions about what bothers the other person.

Imanol, a practitioner of Nonviolent Communication in Spain, told me a story about a relative who moved in with his family when the man's dementia finally made it impossible for him to live on his own. This relative was now in good company, living with people who cared about him and were able to better look after his needs. But what were his needs? He kept wandering around his new house, all day and all night long.

People with dementia are known to wander, often seemingly aimlessly. They may wander from room to room in the house or roam the neighborhood. The wandering may appear crazy and pointless. But if you get interested in where someone is venturing, they may tell you they have a very precise goal—to meet a very particular need. You can help them find a way to fulfill this need, once you know what it is.

Imanol's family began wondering what their relative was searching for. So they paid attention, and one day realized that he was looking for the staircase that would take him to his bedroom upstairs. Except, the house he was now living in was a bungalow. Looking for stairs that were not there kept him busy, but so unsatisfied. Was he looking for his own home, his own place?

Yvonne often told me she wanted to be taken home, even when she was sitting inside her own house. After I took her outside in the wheelchair and asked her to guide me to her home, she settled in. And it wasn't because we had gone anywhere different: we ended up exactly where we had started. I believe it was the connection between us that made her feel at home. I believe that connecting in an empathic way—connecting around real needs—satisfied Yvonne's strong value for independence and provided her with a sense of being understood. I imagine that might feel warm, like a real home would. And I believe that's what Yvonne was really after.

There was a time, though, when Yvonne's family decided

that her own house wasn't a strategy for home that worked for her anymore. Eventually, they moved her to a care home, which she adopted as her residence. Not that she accepted it as her home! Rather, she treated it as her holiday destination. She didn't quite understand what she was doing there, but various clues made her think she was on vacation and staying at a hotel. With all the nice chambermaids and chefs, she found it so much better to be there than at her own house. And it never occurred to her that the vacation went on for rather a long time, because she started each day anew. She was being served everything she needed, so she was pleased. Her needs were met.

This was an unexpected turn of events from the point of view of her family members. They had not expected her to like the care home, especially knowing how independent-minded Yvonne was. But the ways in which needs are met for someone with dementia can be a real surprise. You may find yourself thinking, No wonder I didn't think of this strategy earlier. How could I have imagined this?

Joanne Koenig Coste stresses in her book *Learning to Speak Alzheimer's* that for the emotional well-being of both patients and caregivers, the latter have to acknowledge and relate to patients in their own reality. "Join him [the patient] in his current 'place' or time, no matter when or where that may be, and find joy with him there." When you learn how to be curious about what it is that moves someone, what makes them alive and full of dance and song, you may even be invited to join in!

GUESSING ALOUD

Even when someone with dementia relates well to the world around them, their perception of reality may be significantly different from ours. To understand it, we start with empathic imagination—we guess how they might see, feel, hear, and taste the world around them. And then we use our guesses to learn more about their world and their experience of it.

In guessing what's alive for another person, we needn't worry about getting it wrong. "To play a wrong note is insignificant; to play without passion is inexcusable," said Ludwig van Beethoven. Similarly, guessing incorrectly about how someone feels is insignificant, but not caring how they feel is inexcusable. The passion comes from the heart, both in engaging with music and in engaging with another person. This engagement can move us deeply.

So, begin by caring passionately about your communication with the other person, and focus your imagination on their feelings and needs. How does the current experience, and whatever it is you imagine they perceive, affect them? Then, if you've got language available to make this task easier, inquire with the person directly.

The point is to express genuine interest in their experience. In some cases you may be their voice, their means of expressing themselves. Some people in advanced stages of dementia lose their ability to use language but often not the ability to decipher it. They may be well able to understand what you are saying, and to respond in some way that indicates which of your empathic guesses are accurate, and which guesses express some part of their feelings or needs or requests. And this in itself may be the most connecting experience for you both. As Elizabeth English likes to say, no one can resist being understood.

"I need to see the doctor!" Clare said at times with a sense of urgency. "Why has no one taken me for my medical examination in such a long time? I think it is about time for me to make an appointment."

In fact, Clare had seen her general practitioner earlier that week. So her observation was not *factually* true, but there was something real in it for Clare. Instead of confronting Clare by saying I could prove we'd just been to her doctor, I wondered what she could possibly mean by her complaint. What was she was trying to say?

Once I become sufficiently interested in finding out, I can ask. I can try to guess what matters to Clare at that moment and ask her if my guess is correct. And because I know she lives with dementia, I won't argue with her about her observations and whether they are factually true.

I've learned from my dementia relationships that the concept of dementia allows me more openness toward the other. Paulette Bray-Narai, a certified trainer with the Center for Nonviolent Communication in Australia, whose father has dementia, agreed. She found that the dementia diagnosis brought clarity, especially for herself and her siblings as their father's caregivers. The knowledge helped them to stay present to their father's confused words and actions without needing to defend anyone or argue any mistaken beliefs.

Acknowledge their dementia to yourself, and to them acknowledge their feelings and needs.

In his book *I Am Not Sick, I Don't Need Help!*, Xavier Amador says that listening and empathizing are the most effective tools in reaching the other person who, due to a mental illness, is not on the same page as you. "You will win on the strength of your relationship rather than on the strength of your argument," says Amador.

To connect with someone who has dementia, acknowledge their illness to yourself, and acknowledge their feelings and needs to them. First, choose simple, plain language. Research shows that the simpler the words, the less abstract and more concrete, the more likely it is that the listener will understand us and our intentions. At the back of this book is a list of universal human needs identified by Nonviolent Communication trainers over time. For instance, humans need appreciation, contribution, and inclusion. It's easier to reach someone with dementia if you name their needs not by the abstract idea, such as inclusion, but by naming something close to what you imagine the person wishes to happen. So instead of asking if someone needs inclusion, you might ask if they would like to be a part of the conversation. You might even ask what would help. For example: Would you enjoy people speaking more slowly? Instead of asking if someone longs for contribution, you might ask if they want to help with something.

When you inquire about what matters to someone in language that is easy for them to understand, it may be music to their ears.

EXAMPLES OF DEMENTIA-FRIENDLY EMPATHY

Affection: Would you like a hug? Do you want someone to hold your hand?

Freedom: Do you want to decide by yourself what works for you?

Mourning: Do you want to show how sad you feel? Are you so, so sad?

Participation: Do you want to have a say in what we do? Do you want to be part of what's going on? Would you enjoy people walking slowly?

Respect: Do you want to be cared about? Would you like to be taken into consideration?

(See Appendix B for a more comprehensive list of dementia-friendly language for empathy and guessing needs.)

Second, respect their rhythm. When we are motivated to know what is going on for someone with dementia, we put our attention on their feelings and needs. We reach out to meet them empathically. But sharing one's needs is like opening the doors into private territory, so make sure you remain respectful if they won't let you in. You may not be welcomed—not that day, or at that moment, but your interest in what's going on for them will be noted, and it does matter. Even if the instance is not remembered as a fact, it will be sensed by the heart.

Your interest in what's going on with someone will be noted. Even if the instance is not remembered as a fact, it will be sensed by the heart.

Lastly, bear in mind that with dementia, feelings are more faithful to our shared reality, while memories distort and misrepresent it.

"I haven't seen the doctor for many months now," said Clare. "Why haven't you taken me there?"

She was referring to me—the person who managed her diary and organized a to-do list of all the things that concerned Clare's day-to-day life. I was also the very person who *had* taken her to regular medical appointments.

So when Clare said, "Why has no one taken me for my medical examination in such a long time?" I had to decide how to respond. I wanted to imagine what she might be experiencing and guess what need was important to her right then. I wanted to guess using simple language and be prepared for her to respond in her own time. And I could be pretty sure she wouldn't be easily convinced that she already had her medical appointment that week.

It's often tempting to assume that there is something wrong; like assuming that Clare must have felt sick and that's why she inquires about the doctor. At other times, I expected Clare was worried about the medication prescribed by the very doctor we had just seen.

This left me puzzled. You can see how many assumptions I was making about her original comment. I assumed she was either feeling unwell or annoyed at not receiving enough care and attention. But she hadn't actually said any of those things. Only later did it occur to me to ask her directly about what was on her mind.

"When you say, 'I need to see the doctor!' do you mean to say you are feeling unwell and require medical care?" I asked.

She shook her head in disagreement. "Oh, no. I'm not feeling that bad."

I made a second guess: "So, are you requesting that I take care of you now?"

"No, it is not that. But I may get worse soon. There is something wrong with me and I need to see the doctor."

"Right. I would like to understand, so please bear with me. Do you mean to say that you are troubled because you think something is wrong?" She nodded. "And you would like to see the doctor, hoping he will tell you what is wrong?"

"I can feel something is wrong."

"I'm guessing you would like to understand what's happening to you?"

"The doctor should be able to tell me what's going on."

This was a touching moment when Clare shared with me her longing for understanding and clarity. I realized she did not have any clear memory of any recent visits to her doctor. Even though every effort had been made by the medical professionals to keep Clare informed about her vascular dementia, she lacked an ability to comprehend what was being explained to her while we were there. By the time a day or two had passed, Clare did not remember the visit, let alone what was said. And she was left with a vague recollection about two things: that there was something wrong with her health, and that the doctor had the answer to what it was. The feeling of unease stayed on, while the memories faded away.

As you can see, we would not have got far if we had spent our time trying to establish an accurate observation, then tried to convince Clare she had seen the doctor already. Clare's perception of the situation was not an accurate account of what happened, but it was a direct expression of her need for understanding and clarity. When we connected on the level of her feelings and needs, we were able to meet those needs directly—while respecting what I was willing and prepared to do.

Thereafter, every time we saw a doctor I took time to type everything I could remember from the meeting, in simple language and big font. I left this printed document in a visible place, and Clare often spent hours, literally, studying what it said, occasionally asking me additional questions. This contributed to her sense of understanding. I knew that if I had provided her with this document *before* we connected, and before I guessed her needs empathically, it wouldn't have worked. She would have been fixated on the doctor as the only solution to her problem, and would have continued insisting on a daily basis to see the doctor.

I was willing to take a leap of faith and guess her underlying needs. She wanted to understand herself, and so did I. We shared something special, and when I learned how to receive her needs that way, it became a gift.

Each little gift like this is to be enjoyed while it lasts. Like ice cream, it melts away. But isn't it delicious? Such fleeting joy cannot solve all problems or ease all difficulties, but tasting the sweetness of human needs connects us to each other. All we need to do is to learn how to receive it.

JUST WITNESSING

Receiving what someone has to offer doesn't necessarily require any action from us. We can be there as a heart-witness for them while they connect with themselves. We can help them stay in the moment by being present and interested in their experience. Nothing else.

Melanie Sears, a certified trainer with the Center for Non-violent Communication who once worked as a registered nurse in a behavioral health unit, used to run an empathic support group to provide patients with an opportunity to express and receive empathy, in other words, to recognize and attend to their feelings and needs.

Most of the participants were in advanced stages of dementia and were disoriented, confused, and unable to express themselves clearly. It was as if their inner lives had become foreign, rough, and unfamiliar terrain, where it was easy to lose one's bearings. But one patient, a former psychotherapist, was very articulate and precise in expressing her feelings. Her inner life was familiar ground: she felt at ease in it, completely at home and grounded. She was fluent in describing her inner world.

Melanie found it so easy to relate to this woman—to converse with her about her diagnosis of dementia and connect with her feelings and needs—that she began to wonder whether the diagnosis of dementia was a mistake, an unfortunate misunderstanding.

But when the group was over, Melanie realized the former therapist didn't understand that she was under psychiatric care, and that she was currently a patient in the hospital. She appeared to have no knowledge of where she was, nor the cognitive capacity to comprehend her outer circumstances. Yet she had full capacity to live and express her inner life. Her emotional intelligence made all the difference, making her inner landscape a friendly and familiar place where she could comfortably meet others. And connect.

Most of us haven't developed all the skills a trained psychotherapist would, but each of us—with and without dementia—can become more competent at connecting with our inner life. Even if only through moments of self-reflection.

Although Dory appeared utterly unaware of her brain's condition the majority of the time, every now and then she reflected on her own dementia too. Sometimes I was able to join her while she was paying a visit to her inner land. One such visit took place during her personal skin care treatment, when I helped her rub aloe vera cream onto her very dry skin.

"You know, I never thought it would happen to me," Dory said out loud once, in what appeared to be a response to a reflection that was occupying her mind. Since she said it in my presence, I asked, "What do you mean, Dory?"

"I never thought I would get confused, because my mother never did."

I guessed that by "confused" she meant Alzheimer's, and that the memory of the diagnosis must have surfaced and made Dory wonder what it meant to her. She then told me a little story about her mother and how she remained clear in her mind till the last day of her life. She was never confused.

Then I dared to bring the word *dementia* into the conversation, to be sure that we were talking about what I thought we were talking about. "And how do you notice dementia in yourself?" I asked.

"I sometimes get very confused," Dory said. "But the thing is that I never know when I am confused and when I'm not."

She had not used the words *dementia* or *Alzheimer's*. Rather, *confused* was a more precise and accurate expression for Dory, as it was how she felt the disease in herself. It is an experiential term, and one that expresses an emotion too.

Nothing in this conversation required action from me. But it was an opportunity for me to be actively present and interested in Dory's inner life, and thus support her own connection to it. So I stayed curious about what was going on inside her.

"It sounds like you are feeling pensive, Dory."

"Yes," she said.

Dory was not worried about her illness; at the moment her need was for self-understanding and self-connection. I happened to be a witness. Though she didn't always have the full cognitive ability to process information and situations, she could be clear in herself about feeling confused, and this ironically met her need for clarity, as well as her need for self-empathy. This put her mind at rest, and she spent the rest of that day at ease. At times she said, "Maybe I'm just confused!" and smiled. Not a big deal. At least not that day.

It's possible none of this self-reflection would have taken place if there hadn't been a person there with whom Dory could share. People with dementia are no longer accumulating new memories, but instead, they are integrating what they already know about themselves and the world. Caregivers can enable such integration by simply being present. You can be the person who is eager to hear what's alive for another person. Be a witness to them as they pay attention to their experience.

Carl Rogers, one of the founders of the humanistic approach to psychology, acknowledged that empathic relationships can be formed outside of a therapy room.

Therapeutic relief can take place even if the person listening has no special knowledge of psychology, psychiatry, or medicine. No amount of professional training and academic education is

more worthy than an open heart filled
with empathy for the other.

Caregivers, however, may at any
time feel they've got enough on their
plate, and sometimes their own
self-care will be a priority for their
relationship. In this case, caregivers
might consider finding a professional
who offers therapy sessions suitable for
someone with dementia. "But what's the point of that, since they
won't remember anything anyway?" a friend asked me one day.
Fair enough question, I thought. But it has been my experience that
the point of empathic listening isn't that someone with dementia
remembers the session, but that they feel heard.

The point of empathic listening isn't that someone with dementia remembers the session, but that they feel heard.

Danuta Lipińska, a Polish counselor specializing in aging
and dementia care, shares a similar approach in her book
*Person-Centred Counselling for People With Dementia: Making
Sense of Self*: "It is my belief that men and women living with
dementia must be offered the opportunity to receive professional
counselling if they would like it, to support them in making sense
of their lives, and making sense of themselves in their present
experiencing."

Anyone who cares about someone with dementia can play a
role—in empathic listening, in being a heart-witness. No small
amount of caring attention is ever insignificant.

Tuning In to Anger and Confusion

You know, one of the tragedies of real life
is that there is no background music.

—ANNIE PROULX, *American author*

Outbursts of anger accompany some of the tragic events of almost everyone's life. Anger, anguish, and confusion are loud emotions, which scream and howl to the point that no one can hear the music. When it's not you but a person you care for who is angry, it's very difficult to take in, unless you tune in to what's behind the feelings.

Anger, despair, and anguish are emotions that are inflamed. Any emotion left ignored for long enough will desperately seek attention. It will do what it must to get someone to notice that some needs have gone painfully empty and unfulfilled. An emotion that is ignored long enough will set itself on fire.

Unfulfilled needs are often painful. And we all make the mistake of looking outward for someone or something to blame for our pain. But doing so doesn't fulfill our needs. It doesn't bring us any closer to the real cause of our despair. People angry at dementia proclaim war, and gear themselves up against it. Projecting anger outward—at scientists for not coming up with a cure, at the government for not offering more support, at care services for being inadequate—may prompt you to take collective political action.

But until we address the real cause of our feelings, the suffering will continue to consume us from within. And it will be counterproductive: anger saps rather than strengthens our resources and abilities to do something about dementia.

Blaming ourselves doesn't help in the slightest either. It usually makes things even worse. Angry people who turn their pain inside or attack themselves with self-hatred will slide into the darkness of depression. Directing anger inward in self-hatred is a dead end. Often literally.

When you have your own anger to deal with, the tools in Part Two of this book can help. But what will help you deal with the anger, despair, and confusion expressed by someone with dementia?

UNCOVERING THE NEEDS BEHIND ANGER

Yvonne went in for a general checkup and ended up staying in the hospital much longer than expected. She had encountered very friendly staff, you see, all telling her, "Now be a good girl and sit still" or "Stand up for me, love." Well, Yvonne wouldn't have any of that. After all, she was a lady, she had her pride, and she found this kind of speech that "we're all mates here" infantilizing. She got really, really angry, and then tried to kick the nurse who was helping her. She kicked hard, but blindly, and instead of reaching the person she was aiming for, each time the nurse approached, she kicked out and her leg hit the side of the hospital bed.

She must have done it several times, and with all her force, stoked by anger. This violent expression of anger and anguish left Yvonne with a deep, bleeding wound on her leg. A wound that required even more interactions with nurses and a much longer stay at the hospital, where she continued to be referred to as "love" by strangers.

How often do we hurt ourselves when we express anger unskillfully? When someone expresses explosive emotions violently, both parties get hurt. Often the attacker is in as much pain as the person whom they attack. Indeed, they must be in pain already to have become so angry in the first place.

There is only one reason people with dementia experience anger and other explosive emotions, and it's a very good reason. They are angry because they have beautiful values inside them that demand to be acknowledged, not because they have a short temper. When their needs aren't being met, their anger will remind you. It is your wake-up call.

People with dementia are angry because they have beautiful values inside them not because they have a short temper.

When Yvonne expressed her anger at the nurses for doing things to her that she couldn't comprehend, or talking to her in a manner she found condescending, she was longing—deeply—for clarity and respect. These are needs she had been missing terribly since dementia began to change her cognitive abilities, since she had to rely more and more on others. I am sure the nurses tried to explain what was happening to Yvonne and did not mean to be disrespectful. They knew about her dementia, and to put things plainly, I expect they turned on the childlike speech I have heard so often among medical professionals.

None of that landed well with Yvonne. And so no one's needs were met—not Yvonne's and not the nurses. Needs can't be met if neither party is able to acknowledge them. Fortunately, it's not necessary for both parties to be capable of acknowledging their needs—it's enough if you are able to guess imaginatively what matters to the other person.

Fran's friend Diamantina lived in a residential home, where staff reported her to be "difficult" and to exhibit "challenging behavior." And isn't this exactly what they expect from someone who has Alzheimer's? "Difficult behavior" and "outbursts of anger" are often associated with the illness, in a way that seems to suggest that dementia is the source of the explosive emotions.

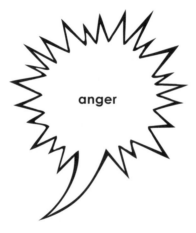

According to Nonviolent Communication, anger is always about desperation to meet needs. Dementia merely makes it harder for someone to communicate those needs.

What needs might have prompted Diamantina's "difficult behavior"? On several occasions Fran witnessed her friend at the table for a meal, and when bits of food remained on her face, one of the staff came around and mechanically wiped Diamantina's face. They did this merely to keep up their care standards, but without any communication. This left Diamantina looking spotless but feeling resentful. She did not welcome people—strangers as far as she was concerned!—keeping up *their* standards by using *her* face! As the situation repeated itself, her resentment grew bigger and bigger, along with her needs for consideration, privacy, and choice.

It was no surprise to Fran that her friend's feelings exploded and resulted in incidents of outburst and conflict. The same staff who labeled Diamantina "uncooperative" were not building a sense of partnership with her, but the exact opposite. This is another example of choosing a strategy whose results are the exact opposite of what is wanted. The staff members who longed for cooperation went about wiping Diamantina's face without her collaboration. How should that bring about any sense of partnership?

It is very common in the human species to confuse a wholesome need in us with the things we want to do to meet that need. In this confusion, this gap between *what* we need and *how* we fulfill that same need, we all—with and without dementia—go seeking things that won't give us what we truly long for.

Professional care providers often try to *make* someone with dementia cooperate. Aggressive solutions such as using restraints or sedatives on patients with dementia—though discouraged in many countries—are still common practice. I see it as a sign of how helpless many dementia care professionals feel. We come up with these unfortunate, misguided ideas when we are not listening to needs carefully enough—our needs or the other person's.

Any caregiver can probably relate to the sense of helplessness when faced with anger from someone they care for. They want the person to be at ease and to calm down. But whether the caregiver achieves this outcome depends on how they go about it.

Strategies such as restraining and sedating, which are meant to be effective, are counterproductive in the end. People with dementia often respond to these strategies by becoming more violent or withdrawing to such an extent that they require even more direct personal assistance and staff time. This violent pacification is a sad contradiction in terms, where "violence" and "peace" appear together. I believe there is no peace where there is violence.

To find more imaginative solutions than violent pacification, it is worth considering that dementia is not responsible for anger or aggression. None of the distress and despair is ever caused by Alzheimer's, nor is any other dementia responsible for someone's cry of anguish. A person who has dementia may have more difficulty expressing their own needs clearly, but their ability to value personal choice and consideration isn't affected by the illness, not even a little bit. People have needs, with or without dementia.

Expressing our needs skillfully means expressing them nonviolently. Nonviolent Communication teaches us to hold on to the awareness that anger and other explosive feelings are caused by our human needs. If someone's language or communication skills are compromised, and we cannot rely on them to clearly recognize and express their needs, we can help by receiving anger skillfully. Because communication is never just what people say, it is also *how* people hear what is said. And the ability to hear anger empathically may be our most powerful nonviolent tool. No one gets hurt.

Of course, we should handle explosive substances with great care, and take the precautions of self-empathy. And we should take extra special care when handling someone who's holding anger in their heart and a sharp tool in their hand.

The ability to hear anger empathically may be our most powerful nonviolent tool.

I once found myself confronted with someone's anger, and though I did not fear for my own safety, I did suspect potential injury. I had found Clare in danger of hurting herself by doing her favorite activity—gardening. We were in the garden, Clare's kingdom, when I saw her holding a pair of pruning shears she had somehow managed to get hold of. I knew that Clare's vision was seriously compromised, and it wasn't often that she was able to zoom in on an object and recognize it for what it was or discern how far it was from her. She had also lost some of her physical coordination skills. So when I saw her with the shears, I was alarmed. I feared for her safety because yes, I questioned her ability to prune plants without harming herself.

I explained this to her and asked whether it would work if I cut the plants for her. Ideally, I tried to encourage Clare's independence as much as possible. But this situation was beyond my comfort zone, so I objected again when I saw Clare leaning forward to give it a go, to try cutting the plants herself before deciding whether to hand the task over to me.

"I will take these shears out of your hand now," I said, "because I don't know how else to protect your health." And I reached out and took the shears away.

Clare's face went white and red at the same time, if you can picture that. I thought I could see anger beaming out of her eyes. She probably wished she could tell me what she thought of me, tell me that I should mind my own business, but when she got emotional her words didn't come easily. As you might imagine, being unable to respond only intensified the heat of the anger she was pouring onto me.

I could have chosen to admit that I was to blame, or to explain to her in many sophisticated words what my reasons were. Instead, in my care that no one should get hurt, I tried my best to guess what was going on for Clare at that very moment. Slowly.

"It looks like you are angry right now," I said. "And I'm guessing that's because you are longing to enjoy activity in the garden." I paused.

"Or maybe you are longing to be able to decide for yourself and choose what you do?"

I did not suggest that she was angry because I took the garden shears out of her hand, nor that she wished I would give the tool back.

Clare looked at me intensely, processing what I said, and then turned around and went into the house. I didn't know what to make of that. I thought the memory of the event had disappeared soon enough, but I also wasn't surprised when Clare gave me the cold shoulder for the rest of the day. Feelings linger, and I could tell I wasn't welcome to inquire about what bothered her.

The next day in the garden, Clare turned to me as if she had just remembered something important. "It is so good what you did the other day," she said.

"You mean taking the pruning shears away?" I asked. "I thought you had been rather irked."

"No, I have been thinking . . ." Claire shook her head. "I love gardening . . . but I need reminding what I can handle."

Dementia makes it impossible for people to do lots of tasks single-handedly anymore. The helping hand of a caregiver is not always welcomed straightaway. At those times the best help you can offer is an attentive ear.

FINDING CLARITY INSIDE CONFUSION

For people living with dementia, confusion is a state even more common than anger. Those with dementia sometimes seem to live in a world from decades ago. They may perceive objects or voices that aren't visible or audible to us, or converse with people we know are long dead. To those of us without dementia, they may seem to have lost touch with reality. Hence some approaches to dementia care emphasize "reorienting them to reality." For example, correcting someone with dementia by saying, There is no alligator in the room, so don't be scared. Or, Now calm down, your father died fifty years ago. He is certainly not shouting at you. These attempts at "reorienting to reality" often feed a person facts from our own sensible world, and they manipulate feelings through commands such as Don't worry, Calm down, or There's no reason to cry.

Reorienting people to reality sounds good to me but what reality are we going to prioritize?

I'm not saying I believe each of us lives in different worlds that are separate and disconnected. I am saying we can choose to reorient ourselves to the reality that is the closest to us and most alive—the reality of our feelings and needs. Most of us—with dementia and without—have lost touch with this reality, with this inner, most immediate world of ours. Instead of demanding that others change their outlook, we could reorient ourselves to our own world of experience.

From this perspective, people with dementia are often way ahead of us. Though they may appear to have lost touch with reality, they often have quite tangible contact with their own inner reality. The sphere that occupies most people—social conventions, facts, figures, and world affairs—means less and less to those with dementia. Their focus changes from being outward-oriented to inward-oriented.

Now, coming into fresh contact with the inner world isn't always the easiest experience. Some people with dementia freak out when they face their own inner land. That's only because it is unfamiliar and they lose their bearings. But with help, they can find their way through this difficult, and at times scary, territory. Empathic communication can be deeply connecting, across any two worlds.

Yvonne didn't take it lightly when she started seeing ghosts. On the nights when these phantoms visited her bedroom, she called for me at the top of her lungs, and frantically shared her worries with me while I held her hand.

"There is something wrong with this house. I'm telling you," she would say. "Go and ring the neighbor. Ask them who lived here before we moved in. I want to know who these people are, these ghostly figures! Can you make them go away?"

Yvonne had never previously believed in ghosts or anything paranormal. But what was normal to her anymore? Now she was convinced the house was cursed. It seemed to be all about the house, that the house was the problem. Or was it? Something was alive for Yvonne that was the reality of her experience.

She looked at me with pleading eyes, waiting for me to rush off and call the neighbor. (It was two o'clock in the morning.)

"Are you scared, Yvonne? Is that why you want to inquire about the house?" I asked.

"I need to know who lived here before us. I wondered why they were selling the house so cheaply at the time, you know . . ."

"So you are anxious because you would like to be able to feel safe here?"

"I want to know whether things will get worse if I stay here any longer."

"Ah, so you would like reassurance that it's safe to stay? Is that right?"

"Yes." She took a breath. "Am I going to be okay?"

"Would you like to hear how I feel in this house?" I asked.

With this question, I asked Yvonne for permission to shift her attention to hearing something from my world. When she nodded, I reoriented myself to my own reality.

"I feel safe and out of harm's way while I'm in this house."

Upon hearing this, Yvonne stroked my hand. She took a deep breath. Perhaps her need for reassurance was fulfilled now, or maybe trust played a bigger part in bringing Yvonne peace of mind. For me, it brought a good night's sleep afterward.

Having dementia brings some people to confront their inner land more closely, perhaps for the first time in a lifetime. Some people find their inner experience to be unfamiliar territory, and at first they lose their bearings.

The awareness, perspective, and skills you are learning in this book, and the dementia relationship you are learning to build, can help provide enough context for people with dementia to make themselves at home. What you have learned can also help them overcome the sense of loneliness they might experience when realizing that each of us has our own world to inhabit.

A dementia relationship, like any other meaningful companionship, is all about meeting each other at the threshold of our worlds. If we stubbornly insist on one reality only, meeting others there may be difficult. If your world has no room for other perceived worlds, you may miss out on the joy of contributing to each other's well-being. I believe that no other person can make us happy, but that happiness comes from fulfilling another's needs and having our needs fulfilled. This is the joy of giving and receiving empathically. The joy of communicating between worlds.

You don't need to believe in anything paranormal to connect with someone who has dementia. You don't have to buy into someone else's idea of the afterlife or believe the stories you hear about ghosts. There is certainly no point in trying to convince someone who may experience hallucinations that they are deluded or wrong in their experience.

You can connect with the authenticity of feelings and needs

instead. As long as you can focus on the reality of needs alive in your heart and the heart of the person you care for, you will have a meeting place. The heart's reality is a genuine reality you can rely on.

This reality is precisely where Kathleen, a Nonviolent Communication trainer, met up with her father. She met him at the doorstep of his world and listened to his needs. "I never felt that I lost my father," said Kathleen. "Despite his dementia."

When he stopped making sense, she understood that he was sens-ing instead. Once he told her that he had recently moved back to Kansas, even though she knew he remained in Colorado, where their conversation was taking place. But she knew he associated Kansas with his family roots, so she sens-itively asked, "Are you excited about moving back to Kansas because that's where your family roots are? Does reconnecting with your family matter to you? Is that what's on your mind? " And he said, "Yes! Yes!" His daughter's empathic presence left him feeling understood and encouraged to share the most meaningful things that took place in his world.

The other person's world isn't so far away that you can't reach them. On the contrary, if you sense what's important for them, you can meet them right there, in that moment. When you listen to what they share with you, focus on what matters to them at that place, at that very moment. What is it that they care about, what is it that feels meaningful right then?

You may not only avoid losing a loved one, but also gain a friend. Melanie Sears, who worked as a nurse at a dementia care home, quickly learned that "reorienting people to reality" wasn't the way to make friends. The routine questions—today's date, the president's name, one's actual age—were obviously too boring to engage with. Some folks choose more fun things to do. One day

Melanie walked into a patient's room and was invited to a private tea party, with imaginary cups, saucers, and cakes. It was rather fun. As Melanie got into her role, she made an excellent guest. The interaction certainly made the patient feel very content, as Melanie's care met their need for companionship and celebration.

Can you imagine this scenario if Melanie had reoriented her patient to the reality of the care home instead? Well, it's clear they would have missed out on a jolly good party.

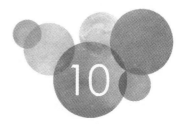

Asking Questions

Every act of memory is to some degree
an act of imagination.

—GERALD EDELMAN, *American biologist*

" What is this Nonviolent Communication?" Olle's mother asked.

Olle, a certified trainer with the Center for Nonviolent Communication who lives in Scandinavia, learned that it didn't help to say, "Don't you remember? I was certified as a trainer in Nonviolent Communication last year. We've talked about it millions of times."

Olle's training in Nonviolent Communication had been a dominant topic in his conversations with his mother for a couple of years. Initially, he interpreted her lack of recollection as an indication that she wasn't listening, or didn't care enough in the first place. Later, when she was diagnosed with dementia, it became clear that his mother had not only forgotten previous conversations, but was genuinely unaware of her memory lapses.

Many people are discouraged when faced with the challenge of how someone's dementia affects their ability to hold a conversation.

Conversation requires more energy, and one quickly learns to be careful about questions. You can't ask everyday questions such as, Don't you remember? or What day is your appointment? or What did the doctor say? The person you're talking to may not recall any of it. Or they may give you one answer, repeated over and over, or instead ask you questions just as repetitive.

I watched Dory get fed up with her friend Beth who also had dementia, saying there was no point in talking to her anymore. As a teenager, I left my great-grandmother's company as soon as I realized she would never move forward with our conversation in the way I expected. I didn't know how to engage with her when ordinary questions such as, What did you do then? didn't work the way they were supposed to. Some approaches to dementia care even advise you to stop confronting people who have dementia with any sort of question—to save them from stress, or the embarrassment of not remembering. Yet without these interactions, conversations may become lifeless or simply boring.

Instead, with empathic presence as our baseline and a few key ideas in mind, we can add some heart-to-heart beat to our daily conversations with people who have dementia. You'll use some imagination, let go of conventions, and explore new conversational areas: landscapes that are unknown to you, but they are exactly where the person with dementia has something to say.

EXPLORING A KALEIDOSCOPE OF MEMORIES

Most of us think of memories as history, facts that are faithfully preserved in our brains. We assume that events happened exactly as we remember them. But our minds are far more creative. We put a spin on everything we remember in a way that is relevant to us—to the "me" that each of us thinks we are. We end up with a collection of memories that are *me*-aningful, that mean something to *me*. Hi-story is made of facts of the world, whereas my me-story is made of facets of myself.

It is worth asking ourselves which story, whether objective history or subjective me-story, we go for? Which one has more life in it? Do we live to collect memories, or to experience life? One could say that the collection basket of someone with dementia has a hole in it and their memorabilia are leaking out, but they are not any less capable of experiencing life than they have ever been.

> *Do we live to collect memories, or to experience life?*

By the time you are old enough to read this book, but not too old yet, you have lived for at least seven thousand days. By the time you are in your sixties, you will have lived twenty-two thousand days. That's an awful lot of days to remember. And none of us remembers every single one of them, do we? Do you remember what you did on your three-thousandth day, not long after you turned eight years old? Probably not, unless something significant happened on that day.

It's not because we have dementia that we don't remember each day. We forget most of our days because it's not necessary to remember them all. Not all are meaningful to our me-story. Do you remember the license plate number of the car you were driving behind yesterday, or what you had for lunch on Tuesday exactly two months ago? By sheer necessity, we edit out days, events, names, and all sorts of other data. Like modern-day hard drives, our brains have limited capacity for storage. We successively get rid of caches of memory from our everyday lives.

Yet there are things we will never forget. And they are not what you might predict you will always remember. We remember significant events and bits of information, and occasionally something random. Our brains seem to have minds of their own, and they play with memories. But generally, we keep in front of our minds the events and information that make us who we are, at least in our own eyes.

This is no different from someone who lives with dementia. People with dementia remember things which are significant to them in some way, that make them who they think they are. The process of editing our memories, however, remains mysterious. You might indeed wonder whether certain events or facts were removed at random or were simply not that significant to the person.

I run workshops for members of the general public who want to learn something about memory and dementia. Henry was a participant in one of these events, a man in his sixties with lots of personal history.

I asked him to tell his life story three times, in three minutes or less each time, and each time using different events to illustrate his history. It was an interesting exercise for him, especially because of the personal reflection that followed. Henry reflected afterward on what he had not mentioned in his three life stories and was completely astonished when he realized he had not mentioned his two grown children in any of his accounts. What was that about? Did it mean something?

It is not uncommon for people living with dementia to lose track of any memory of having children, a spouse, or siblings. Any close relationship is in danger of being edited out—or perhaps recycled, so that the husband entering the room is taken for a father or a son. These relationships may not have been insignificant, but quite the opposite. As Philip Roth wrote in *American Pastoral*, "We don't just forget things because they don't matter but also forget things because they matter too much. . . . Each of us remembers and forgets in a pattern whose labyrinthine windings are an identification mark no less distinctive than a fingerprint."

Regardless of the reason, or the algorithm, that determines which memories stay on, some memories always last, even through advanced stages of dementia. I call these memories a person's me-story. My experience is that these stories are associated with the person's sense of self—who they think they are and what makes them *them*. No matter how closely you are related to someone, by definition their me-stories are never about you. They are about them.

These stories are precious—they are precious to the person with dementia, and they may become precious to you too. You may learn things about the person from their own perspective, from within their inner world. If you never knew someone before they got dementia, these stories are a way to get to know them. And even if you've known someone for a long time, or all your life, their core stories will enable you to get to know them from within.

I still remember the time I was introduced to the home situation of Yvonne, who was a new client at the time. When I inquired about her story, one of her long-term, live-in caregivers said, "You should ask Yvonne herself. She would love to tell you the story of her life." Now I always ask to hear it from the horse's mouth. Because a me-story is their story to tell, in exactly the way they want to.

Dementia often frees people from social constraints: they may be much more honest, and often much funnier, than before. They have most likely forgotten who they were supposed to be. And who you are too.

"Do you remember me?" was a question that Fran used to ask.

She used this question to greet her friend Diamantina, in hopes it would bring some memories back. Instead, it seemed to make

Diamantina a little uncomfortable. She clearly didn't recognize Fran from her appearance alone.

It's easy in situations like these to misinterpret lack of recognition as lack of care and to think: You would remember me, if this relationship mattered to you as it does to me.

Over time, Fran learned that it worked much better for their relationship if she, after knocking first, walked into Diamantina's room *as a friend* and made herself at home. Through her friendly behavior and her sense of ease in their private room, she gave Diamantina clues that *they must be friends*. By bringing ease into the room, Fran could then connect with her friend. This was a revelation to Fran, who found she could now trust their connection and not worry so much about memories.

Diamantina is now convinced that Fran is one of the residents of the care home. She describes Fran as "a dear, friendly soul" and "a fellow resident." This meets Fran's need for connection, which is the healing factor for their relationship.

If you can no longer rely on the template from your previous relationship, you will need to get to know each other anew. You both have lots to learn about the person you share a dementia relationship with. Who is this person? When you use empathy to be curious, you can forget the past the way you remember it and instead learn the stories that are significant to the person you care for.

Dementia is often said to be about memory loss. But no matter how many dates, facts, names, and faces have been forgotten, there's one area that often goes untouched: that saved memory zone is someone's me-story. That is where their truth lies, where they feel most confident and at home, and where they are willing to meet new people. If you want to connect with someone who has dementia, meet them there.

In this place, they are the authority. The me-story is not a collection of facts—not a true, verifiable account of events. It is a "me" version of it, which is precisely what makes the me-story so personal. The person who shares with you their me-story allows you into their intimate world, where things makes sense internally, not externally. It is a great privilege. You do not learn about the facts of someone's life as much as you learn about the meaning of their life events and what impact they had.

Remember the delight in my Grandma Maria's eyes when I asked her about her immediate family? She knew her me-story well, even if it was the last story she could remember. And this very story defined for herself who she was: she was a person whose family moved up North, and she wanted to go and visit them there.

ASKING NEW QUESTIONS ABOUT OLD STORIES

Repetition in a dementia relationship tends to bother only one party. Most people who have dementia don't have a problem with repeating the same comment, phrase, or question multiple times. In a similar fashion, the person with dementia doesn't have a problem wearing their underwear on top of their clothing. If you are bothered by these things, then you need to learn how to make it work for you. You can learn to see the other person's tendency to repeat themselves as an act of kindness. They are giving you another chance to connect, and one more after that.

"So, dear, what did you do during the war?" Yvonne asked me.

A few weeks earlier, Yvonne had a bad injury, and in her recovery, she became more interested in conversing. At the time, she was approaching her hundredth birthday, and the year we met was exactly seventy-three years after the Second World War broke out in Europe. We were sitting in her living room, surrounded by objects that looked to me like carefully arranged museum artifacts. The environment was reminiscent of the times of war, so in this sense, her question was appropriate to the setting. "What did you do during the war?" is a question that acquaintances asked one another at that time in history.

So I took the question to be her way of getting to know me. I knew about the war from school, from books and movies, and occasionally I heard snapshots of war stories from my grandparents who were eyewitnesses in Poland. But for me, the war belonged to the distant past. It was almost surreal—a terrible shadow of the past that cast its darkness upon the modern world I was born into. So if I am asked what I did during the war, I say I've got nothing to do with the war. Thankfully, it is not part of my life, and there isn't much more to be said on that topic.

In our very first conversation when Yvonne asked, "So, dear, what did you do during the war?" I answered, "Well, I wasn't born yet."

"Oh, yes. Of course—you are so young, I've forgotten," said Yvonne. "So what about your parents?"

"My parents weren't born either. They were born in the 1950s, so ten years after the war ended."

"Goodness, you are a child! It is a surprise that you can walk!"

That was sarcastic. I could hear it in her tone of voice. And I could see that Yvonne had lost interest in the conversation. She turned her head away from me, reached for the remote control, and turned on the television. It was almost a theatrical gesture. She wanted to switch me off by changing the channel from me—a person talking nonsense—to another talking head. So that's where our conversation stopped, at least the first three or four times.

I sometimes added that Yvonne was a generation older than my grandparents. My grandparents were born only a couple of years before the war broke out. But this information didn't make our conversation go any better.

Thankfully, Yvonne kindly gave me many more opportunities to practice my response, and I got better at it each time. It happened on different occasions, during different times of day, but always started with the same question: "What did you do during the war?" Each time she asked I had an opportunity to experiment with different replies and therefore experience different outcomes.

Part of me found it funny that I needed to explain how I hadn't taken part in a war that happened two generations before I was born, and part of me found it grotesque. Whereas for Yvonne, it was a serious inquiry and my answers were pure nonsense. We were clearly not on the same page. In order for my answers to make sense, she had to get her head around the fact that the year was 2012, and that she was ninety-seven years old.

These were facts in the so-called objective world, the world in which the objects in her living room were more than seventy years old. But I realized that Yvonne didn't think she was that old; she hadn't aged in the same way the objects in her home had aged. From comments she made on several occasions, I determined that she thought she was in her late thirties. She aged in her own way, and as far as she was concerned, if you wanted to meet her, you had to meet her as a thirty-year-old woman.

For her the war was relevant, a hot topic that everyone discussed, and all current news was about the war. In her world, the war had just happened, as if it was yesterday. After many, many attempts at responding appropriately, one day I realized I had completely misunderstood her question! It dawned on me that her question about what I did during the war didn't mean she wanted to hear about *me*, but instead it meant: Would you like to hear what I did during the war?

She told me about volunteering to be on the night watch during the London bombings. She would sit on the roof of the Ritz Hotel, the highest point in the city they could access at that time, and observe the night sky in case she or her companions caught a glimpse of the enemy's air force. If they did, they would warn the community to go to the shelters. She told me this not as a terrifying story, but as an exciting and delicious experience—partly because in exchange for her service, she and the other night watch volunteers received free food from the finest hotel restaurant in the country.

She was right in the midst of the war, in the heart of the country's capital, being brave, daring, and courageous. She did not have a driver's license, but she could drive, and London needed drivers. So she offered her service as an ambulance driver, and she once delivered a patient to the hospital through the bombed streets of the city while the doctor on board was giving the patient a heart massage. They saved his life.

Yvonne's mother, meanwhile, provided shelter at their home for countless Polish soldiers who gathered in the cellar each evening to sing Polish songs. Yvonne joined them at times, and they had a jolly good time together. Who knows, maybe my great-grandfather Antoni, whose army service took him to Britain, was among these soldiers! I never met him, as he never reunited with his family in Poland. He eventually settled and died in Wales, not far from where I live now. I discovered his grave no less than fifty years after his death. But maybe Yvonne knew him. Maybe our lives were mysteriously interwoven throughout time and history.

When I was in her world as a polite visitor, she was generous with her stories and tales. When we were connected in this way, I as a visitor, she as the host, I could ask her all sorts of questions, and she felt confident and utterly competent to answer them.

For someone with dementia, questions are neither frightening nor confrontational if you inquire about their world. Yvonne knew everything there was to know in her own world. Literally. And as my friend Ian Mackenzie likes to say, "Open questions create the habit of openness." Questions that open a conversation further are questions like: What was that like? Was it fun? Wasn't it scary? Will you tell me more?

For someone with dementia, questions are not frightening if you inquire about their world.

Removing distractions, like background noise or television, also helps when talking to someone with dementia. And keeping to one topic at a time makes it easier for them to follow what you are asking about. Simplify as much as possible. Simplicity often brings depth.

I learned all this after finally getting the message that it was time to explore Yvonne's memories, by her sharing them with me. Little did I know, initially, that this treasure of memories was hidden behind the repetitive question, "What did you do during the war?"

Hearing Yvonne ask me the same question repeatedly was, in the end, so helpful for me. People without dementia learn through repetition, by trying again and again. It is a gift when those with dementia bring up a question, comment, or phrase repeatedly—so that we can explore what to do with it. As the philosopher and poet Criss Jami wrote in *Healology*: "In this repetition manifests one's ability to go on experiencing again the very same thing from a different perspective and in a brand-new light."

Being able to see the same thing from a new perspective is key in a dementia relationship. How often do we catch ourselves giving the *same* response when confronted with the *same* comment, such as: I want to call the police, or I need to get my car back, or Take me home? Do we find ourselves repeating the response or reacting always in the same, habitual way? If so, then we are dealing with double repetitiveness—that of the person with dementia, and that of the person without dementia who is set in their own habits.

Hearing the same comments repeatedly may at times trigger us—in the sense that the comment touches on a sensitive and irritable spot inside us. This can happen for a few reasons. The main reason is that when people who don't have dementia repeat themselves, it usually means they didn't feel heard the first time, or they are being insistent and trying to get their message across. This type of repetition is intentional, and we understand that. So it can be hard for us not to interpret the repetitive remarks of someone with dementia as deliberate. And yet, when you think about it, in a dementia relationship, we can be almost 100 percent sure that the person with dementia has zero recollection of repeating themselves. For them, it's the first time they've said it, and it's therefore quite fresh. To respond to their world, we need to be playful and make sure our responses don't get stale.

Try it, and see what happens. Next time you can try again. And again. And one more time after that. It is not that eventually you will hit upon the only one right response. The right response in these situations is a spontaneous one.

This is a useful approach as long as you can find the fun or lesson in it. But sometimes a repetitive question will be a trigger for us instead to connect with ourselves empathically.

Both of Kathleen Macferran's parents had dementia, and they often called her with the same news, each time enthusiastically sharing something positive they had experienced. For Kathleen, the news wasn't new, but the joy was fresh each time. And it continued to be a joy until Kathleen got breast cancer, and had to undergo a serious but successful operation. For weeks afterward, her mother's regular phone call resulted in the same conversation:

"How are you, dear?"

"I'm well, recovering slowly."

"Recovering? Recovering from what? What is the matter, dear?"

"Mum, I have undergone a major operation."

"Have you? Why didn't you tell me before?"

And because Kathleen's mother didn't recall any details, let alone the fact that her daughter had been ill, Kathleen had to retell the story of her condition each time.

It wasn't fun. It was painful. It was painful to accept that her own mother couldn't retain the knowledge of such a massive, life-changing experience for her genuinely beloved daughter. It was hard to see love and care in the repetitive forgetting which seemed so uncaring and lacking in interest. During her empathic self-care, Kathleen realized that having a choice about how and when to talk about her illness mattered to her.

Having owned this need for choice, Kathleen decided she would like to remind her mother of this key fact in her daughter's life. She wrote a message on a piece of paper: "Kathleen has had major surgery. But she is doing great now." She placed the message by her mother's phone. The painful, repetitive conversations stopped. This simple strategy saved Kathleen the torture of continually retelling the story of her illness. And it probably saved her mother a lot of embarrassment and distress as well.

Writing down the answers to questions you know will be coming, and which you are not able to enjoy answering, may be a respectful solution that satisfies everyone's needs. Matthew, a Nonviolent Communication practitioner from California, also experienced the power of answering questions in this way. When a friend with dementia returned home after a traumatic hospitalization, Matthew found her repeating the same questions over and over in a loop. Appearing agitated and scared and very frustrated, she was unable to assimilate any answers she was given. Matthew carefully wrote down all of her questions, each followed by a brief answer. When he presented his friend with this piece of paper that reflected and addressed all her worries, she instantly relaxed. She settled down and studied the paper.

When our intentions, values, and needs match our strategy, sometimes connection can indeed be mediated through the phone or on paper. Other times, including in advanced stages of the disease, we will increasingly rely on more direct and immediate ways of meeting the people we care for. Staying in touch with them and sustaining a sense of connection is possible even when words are no longer of help.

Staying in Touch

Do not speak unless you can improve on the silence.

—ANTHONY DE MELLO, *Jesuit priest*

The dictionary defines communication as an exchange of information. Nonviolent Communication defines it as an exchange that brings about connection. Nonviolent means of communication are less like delivering parcels of information and more like journeying to meet someone in person.

Nonviolent Communication serves dementia relationships so well because communication in a dementia relationship is about meeting the other person where they are. The focus is not on facts and accounts of factual situations or exchanges of information; it is simply about connection.

This type of connection does not mean using simplistic or superficial ways of talking. It doesn't necessarily mean talking at all. Connection is the inner bond that draws one person to another, not words, as Rumi said. So it is important not to get lost in words. We may then be able to find one another quicker.

A lot could be said about the importance of silence in a human relationship. Many significant life events happen without much talking: birth (both giving birth and being born), first steps walking, kissing, and smiling at one another. And the most significant, strongest experiences in life tend to leave us speechless. And touched.

This chapter is about three things you can use instead of words as means for connection: presence, music, and touch.

PRACTICING INTER-PRESENCE

One day my husband, Scott, and I visited a friend of ours who lived in a residential home. Ed had rapidly progressing dementia. I am sure he didn't recognize either of us as we came into his room, yet he appeared welcoming. The three of us sat down, and I made an attempt to get a conversation going. I asked Ed how things were, and how his meditation was going (since I knew he was a keen meditator).

Ed had a go at answering: it seemed like he had words on the tip of his tongue, and he was patiently waiting until they came out. The silence in the room was the kind that one expects to be broken, like a glass dish that has a crack, everyone assuming it will give, but instead it holds on for yet another minute, and one more after that. Ed stared at the carpet as if not wanting to startle the words that seemed to have lost their way. I patiently waited. Scott was simply present. The clock ticked, and at some point, Ed relaxed his gaze and sat back.

Scott caught Ed's eye and said, "Have they gone for good?"

"Yep," came a quick reply from our friend, admitting that he had lost sight of his skittish words.

So that's that, I thought, with a little embarrassment, I admit. I thought it might be a better idea to chat with the staff to find out how Ed was doing generally. I excused myself, and left the men behind.

When I came back after chatting with a care worker and entered the room, Ed looked surprised to see me. He may well have forgotten seeing me fifteen minutes earlier. With a shadow of uncertainty on his face, he looked to Scott for reassurance, as if asking: Is it okay for this stranger to come in? Scott's relaxed expression told him that everything was fine; she's a friend. And so Ed welcomed me in again and pointed to the place where I could sit.

I sat down and inquired whether they had sat in silence those several minutes I was out, and indeed that was the case. They seemed to have done nothing while I was out, but they had woven connection out of the thin air of silence. Somehow Scott's relaxed presence—his comfort with a silence he did not seek to break, or challenge, or wish to be any different than it was—made a connection. Without inter-action, they enjoyed inter-presence.

I saw this trust that had been built when Ed turned to Scott as a stranger, me, walked into the room. Scott was now included in Ed's inner circle.

It may have been the very first time Scott had met anyone affected by dementia, and yet I was humbled by his beautiful intuition for making connection through silence.

SHARING MUSIC AS EMPATHY TO OUR EARS

When I first met Yvonne, she was wrapped up in blankets, sitting in her wheelchair, and apparently sinking into oblivion and numbness. Or rather, I should say that's how I first saw her, because it was hardly a case of meeting one another. Her eyes were closed and she was unresponsive to anything I said. Her upright position gave me reason to believe she wasn't asleep, and yet she seemed even less present than someone in deep slumber.

I wanted to meet her, but could not do so by saying hello, nor through eye contact. Touch felt inappropriate, as I had no way to tell whether she would welcome it or not. So I tried to find a different way of getting to know her.

Over the course of twelve hours, while Yvonne remained immobile, I looked around her room, and eventually saw a set of old cassette tapes. After some determined hunting around the house, I located an old tape recorder. And I broke the silence with a recording of piano jazz music from the sixties. As sound took over the room, I sat back and began to know Yvonne a little. When a single tear ran down her cheek, that tear carried more meaning than hours of conversation. Though it was another few days before we had our first verbal exchange, this is how I truly met Yvonne. As Victor Hugo said, music expresses that which cannot be put into words and that which cannot remain silent.

Music provides a kind of opening for many people who live with dementia. Some, like Yvonne, open their hearts at the sound of their favorite piano music, others open their mouths upon hearing well-known songs. Some people with profound loss of language can still sing, and even memorize activities or events through singing. For Clare, who struggled with speech due to frequently escaping words, singing was a breath of fresh air, a way to be fluent. I discovered this one Christmas evening when I sang her the carol "Silent Night." She joined me with such delight and surprise—that she not only knew all the words, but that they came out uninterrupted. By then we both were singing, and it turned out to be not a silent night after all.

PRONOUNCING TOUCH

If you haven't experienced much touch in your dementia relationship thus far, now might be a good time to introduce it. Like trust, touch is something you need to establish; you cannot expect it to happen overnight. To develop trust, you let the other person know over time that their needs matter to you. Touch can be a vehicle to deliver this message. Touch can communicate reassurance, support, tenderness, empathy, love, and understanding—as well as your own trust in the other person and your relationship.

By touch, I mean gently placing your hand on the other person's shoulder, or their back, or their hand. It is best introduced in small steps—continuously and consistently. You need to sense your way at first, see what feels appropriate, and what kind of touch they respond to in the way you intended. Touch can also mean sitting in very close proximity to someone, while respecting their private space. In this way you communicate that you are within their close circle; you are family or familiar. It is probably no coincidence that both words share the same root, from the Latin word *familia*. You imply you are on their side.

Because of Clare's compromised vision, touch was a way for me to say: I am here. I am with you. With Yvonne, I held her hand to hold her attention when I wanted to deliver a message to her. With Gordon, I held his arm to help him reorient himself whenever he lost his bearings; I didn't offer touch to him in any other situations. Similarly, Dory welcomed having my arm whenever we went for a walk, to help her with balance. She didn't necessarily respond to touch while we were talking, though she appreciated gentle stroking of her arm when she was distressed.

Ruth, a Nonviolent Communication practitioner, had never had a tactile relationship with her mother, Jane. Their whole family did not hug or connect in this way. But later, Ruth learned the value of touch from her husband; he taught her the importance of holding hands and hugging. She then realized the lack of touch between her parents. After Jane developed dementia and was living in a care home, Ruth often visited, and in Jane's room, reassuring touch and occasional hugs began to be part of their relationship. But one day, when Ruth was with Jane at a hospital appointment, Ruth thought her mother seemed ill at ease, so she put her hand on Jane's arm to offer reassurance. Jane reacted instantly, pulling away with a shudder. When it happened again on a similar occasion, Ruth sensed that her mother made a distinction between public and private: what was okay and even welcomed in her room was not okay, not wanted in public.

Or there might have been other explanations. Maybe their connection, their trust, had not yet developed sufficiently. Also, when people want to stress their independence, they may not welcome touch. Maybe Jane was communicating: I am not a child, I don't need you to hold my hand.

I have worked with people who had dementia and didn't have a clue who I was and didn't remember ever meeting me before, but as soon as I made physical contact with them, they seemed to relax. As if their body remembered me, not their eyes or ears. The sensation of touch may be more memorable and meaningful than someone's visual appearance or the sound of their voice, let alone dry facts. In his book, *Living Without Regret*, Arnaud Maitland reflects on the condition of his fading mother in the following words:

"When doing stops and knowing fails, being remains. As long as there is being, we can make contact. The contact from being to being connects us all and is ever-present, always available. . . . My mother's being, even when mental direction evaporated, was still capable of seeing, hearing, and—especially—sensing."

In the advanced stages of dementia, touch can be your lifeline, your heart-to-heart communication. It is a way to be with each other, a way to say I love you, I am here for you, and I care. These are some of the most important messages one human being can communicate to another, and they can be said without words. Connection outgrows language, and can be translated into silence, presence, and touch.

Experiencing Vulnerability

The heaven I gained from knowing God is this inevitability,
... that, no matter what the hell is going on, if we
get to this level of connection with each other ...
it's inevitable that we will enjoy giving and
we'll give back to life.

—MARSHALL B. ROSENBERG, *American peacemaker*

My Granny Irena, who had been a caregiver for so many years to her mother, died just a few years after we lost Grandma Maria.

I was with my Granny when she was dying. I was a witness to her last breaths. I was twenty-three years old, and the way she looked at me on her deathbed will stay with me for the rest of my life. She was vulnerable and frightened. I didn't know how to help her then. But I made a promise that I would find a way to help that would bring connection and peace.

The time of dying prompts us to address the most profound, and equally the most frightening, questions in life. What is the meaning of life? Is death the end? When we try, as we often do, to close these questions with definite answers, we are trying to shut down our fear. We fear being vulnerable in the face of the unknown. But as Danuta Lipińska, a Polish dementia counselor, says, "This tangible vulnerability, this disarming openness and honesty, are also home to the sacred and spiritual."

Over time I have experienced vulnerability as the most connecting factor in building meaningful relationships. Witnessing my Granny's uneasy passing away is when it started dawning on me that perhaps being vulnerable isn't a weakness but a strength. That it is possible to be vulnerable and fearless at the same time. Because we can trust our connection with each other, which will only grow in strength when we are open and sensitive—be it in living or in dying.

The Buddhist teacher Lama Shenpen Hookham has made it her life's mission to bring to our awareness just how deep our connections with others can go. Because the people we are in relationship with are part of the very fabric, the very essence, of our being. Our relationships can become something that we can trust, something that we can rely on. Especially when we commit to cultivating wholeness and wholesomeness within each and every one of us.

I have taken caregiving as my spiritual practice to put these ideals into practice. To live them through helping relationship. As Ram Dass and Paul Gorham say in the book *How Can I Help? Emotional Support and Spiritual Inspiration for Those Who Care for Others*, "The experience of helping, turns out to be what most spiritual traditions define as the fundamental issue of life itself. Awakening from our sense of separateness is what we are called to do in all things."

It was the promise I gave to my Granny Irena that fueled my quest for awakening. I feel that our connection never died, and it continues giving back to life. It inspired me to write this book. And I will be eternally grateful to my Granny for this connection we share.

Expressing Gratitude
Without a Tail

Gratitude unlocks the fullness of life. . . .
Gratitude makes sense of our past,
brings peace for today, and creates
a vision for tomorrow.

—MELODY BEATTIE, *American author*

"You sound like you would wish dementia on everyone!" Veronica's sister once said to her.

Veronica had been practicing Nonviolent Communication with her mother, Gertrude, who had dementia. Somehow the change that dementia brought into their lives, accompanied by the Nonviolent Communication skills that Veronica was able to put into use, brought the two women together. For the first time in their lives, certainly for the first time since Veronica went to boarding school at age five, they were enjoying a relationship of closeness, mutual understanding, and humor.

Mysteriously, dementia heightened Gertrude's appreciation of beauty. She often said, "But look! Look! Isn't that beautiful?" As if finally, at the age of ninety-six, she could see the quality of beauty as vividly as never before.

Veronica found it very inspiring to witness this stage of her mother's life. Gertude appeared more alive than in her younger years, despite her dementia, wobbly balance, and inflamed feet. Even while talking to me about her mother, now held in loving memory, Veronica said she felt her heart swell with gratitude. She rejoiced at the relationship she had finally experienced with her parent. "It's as if dementia created a new window of communication for us," Veronica said.

For Veronica and her mother, dementia brought wholesomeness into their relationship. For them, as for many other people I know, the illness challenged their ordinary ways of interacting. The deterioration of language, perception, and memory that is common to dementia limits communication, but it can also paradoxically open up opportunities to go deeper with the communication that is left. It can allow us to express to each other something ungraspable, yet deeply touching.

"It's not like I wish the illness on anyone. That's not what I mean," clarified Veronica. "Though the dementia did allow me and my mother to have a deepening intimacy, and moments of playfulness, humor, and ease in expressing unconditional love. I just wish everyone could have that experience of a restored relationship, as I did."

I too have been grateful for my experience with dementia. It has brought things into perspective, focused me on wholeness, connected me to wholesomeness, and committed me to life.

Gratitude is available to all caregivers, and it can be expressed to the person with dementia, but also to yourself. What is it that you appreciate in the person you care for? And in yourself—what are you grateful for?

Dogs have a handy instrument for expressing their gratitude, joy, or appreciation—their tail. As poet W.H. Auden once remarked, "In times of joy, all of us wished we possessed a tail we could wag." We humans, however, have to express our gratitude through other means. Words of gratitude are a start, and add a great deal to a dementia relationship. Yet gratitude itself is not only about words. It is primarily about the experience.

Nonviolent Communication encourages people to express appreciation as celebration—a celebration of life. The experience of appreciation can be thrilling and enthusiastic when addressing the living, or calm and poignant when accompanying the dying. But gratitude lasts longer than any passing emotion. It is a quality of being thankful. You can continue to be grateful for your dementia relationship long after it is over. There is no time limit to this undying connection you have made with another person.

ACKNOWLEDGMENTS

This book is a fruit of my reflections on dementia and my process of making sense of my and other people's experiences. But the underlying ideas on which this work rests were fundamentally influenced by two great pioneers in their own fields: Marshall B. Rosenberg and Lama Shenpen Hookham.

Marshall Rosenberg I have met only indirectly, through his Nonviolent Communication legacy. I learned the process of Nonviolent Communication from CNVC certified trainers including Elizabeth English, Bridget Belgrave, and Gina Lawrie. Certified trainers Kirsten Kristensen, Kathleen Macferran, and Melanie Sears also helped make this book a reality—by loving the idea and by sharing with me their own experiences with dementia.

I would never have heard about Nonviolent Communication if not for Lama Shenpen Hookham. Her commitment to finding and promoting what's real and authentic has been a lifelong inspiration illuminating my path. I have had the good fortune to work closely with her for many years. Her Living the Awakened Heart training, available online, is a big part of my life, and the community of those committed to awakening hearts (The Awakened Heart Sangha) played a vital role in supporting me during the process of writing this book. I would like to thank especially Tara Anne Dew, whose continued generosity cannot be described in words.

This book would not exist without my clients. I have made every effort to maintain the confidentiality and anonymity of my clients with dementia, while remaining true to the spirit of the stories told. All their names, and some personal details, have been changed. I remain so grateful to every one of them for welcoming me into their lives and giving me many opportunities to learn and reflect.

I am also thankful to the caregivers from whom I learned many valuable skills and attitudes, including especially Hannah Wisby, Meave Rowlands, and Edyta Wańkowicz.

We caregivers have Tom Kitwood to thank for his work on person-centered dementia care, and for stressing the role that relationship plays in such care. My personal thanks go to Professor Bob Woods, from the Dementia Services Development Centre at Bangor University in Wales, who has continued with Kitwood's school of thought and who contributed the foreword to this book.

Alzheimer's Society is an organization I value for their unceasing work to raise awareness about dementia in the United Kingdom and beyond, and I've found that what I learned from them about approaching people with dementia is in many ways in harmony with the principles of Nonviolent Communication.

I want to thank Meiji Stewart and PuddleDancer Press, who jumped at the very concept of this book, well before the manuscript was completed.

I am also full of appreciation for my editors. In the early stages, Silvia Rose was my gentle companion in writing. Rachel Edwards joined me in the intermediate stage, providing so much warmth, understanding, and encouragement that the work just carried on. Next I met Kyra Freestar from Tandem Editing LLC, with her wealth of experience, skill, and empathy. She took me not just to another stage of writing, but to another level altogether.

A big chunk of gratitude goes to those who contributed to this book by sharing with me their experience of caregiving, among them Alexandra Wilson, Alvaro Embid, Gert Ceville-Danielsen, Jan Parker, Kate Forster, Katie Morrow, Montse Monereo, Paulette Bray-Narai, Robert Gwyn Davin, and others who chose to remain anonymous. Thank you for your trust.

I would like to acknowledge my dear friends who have been particularly affected by my unavailability as I worked on this project but who continued to support me, especially Elizabeth Elliot, Kasia Kulbowska, Five and Kathy Cram, Vicky and John Hope-Robinson, Sarah Leach, Olga Witkowska, Gabriele Reifenberg and others, including Idalia Smyczynska from kilku.com.

Special thanks go to another very dear friend, Jonathan Shaw, for suggesting I add the word *together* to the title of this book. To Professor Krzysztof Kosior, for his never-ending encouragement to be creative. To Elaine Ward, and my other counseling tutors, for teaching me a person-centered way. I would like to thank my family, especially Melania Mielnik, as well as my husband's relatives, including Michael and Teresa Morrison.

My husband, Scott Smith, was within earshot almost the entire time it took me to write this book. He was listening and looking out for my needs throughout this process, and I felt both heard and seen. My needs were met.

Resources for Dementia and Nonviolent Communication

Alzheimer's and Dementia

Alzheimer's Association (United States of America):
https://alz.org/

Alzheimer's Society (United Kingdom):
https://www.alzheimers.org.uk

Online dementia learning courses:
www.scie.org.uk/e-learning/dementia

Nonviolent Communication

Center for Nonviolent Communication: www.CNVC.org

Online Nonviolent Communication training courses:
https://nvctraining.com/

PuddleDancer Press: www.nonviolentcommunication.com

Dementia-Friendly Empathy

Affection: Would you like a hug? Do you want someone to hold your hand?

Appreciation: Do you want to know if I enjoyed what you did?

Authenticity: Do you want to say or do what's really in your heart? Do you want to share what's true for you?

Autonomy: Would you like to choose what to do?

Care: Do you want to know that I care? Would you like help with this?

Clarity: Would you like to understand what's happening?

Companionship: Would you like some company? Would you enjoy someone sitting next to you?

Compassion: Would you like to know that others have a sense of how hard this is for you?

Competence/Effectiveness: Do you want to be able to do what you want? Do you wish things would turn out more like you plan them?

Consistency: Do you want to be able to count on things going a certain way every time? Do you want people to do what they say they'll do?

Contribution: Would you like to be able to help?

Cooperation: Do you want everyone to work together as a team?

Creativity: Do you want to explore what you are able to make? Do you want to express yourself with music (art, crafts, dance)?

Equality/Fairness: Do you want everyone to matter?

Freedom: Do you want to decide by yourself what works for you?

Honesty: Do you want to trust that people say what is true for them?

Inclusion: Would you like to be a part of what's happening? Would you enjoy people speaking slowly?

Mattering: Do you want to know that you matter? Would you like to know that I care about what you need?

Meaning: Would you like to do things that are important to you?

Mourning: Do you want to show how sad you feel?

Mutuality: Do you want everyone to help one another?

Order: Do you want to find things easily? Do you want to know what's going on around you?

Participation: Do you want to have a say in what we do? Do you want to be part of what's going on? Would you enjoy people walking slowly?

Peace: Do you want a quiet (calm, easy) time?

Play: Do you want to have fun? Do you want to do what you feel like doing?

Predictability: Would you like to know what to expect?

Purpose: Do you want to know what this is for? Would you like to know where we are going?

Respect: Do you want to be cared about? Would you like to be taken into consideration?

Safety/Security: Do you want to know that you will be okay? Would you like to be safe?

Stimulation: Are you looking for fun or something new to do? Do you want to have an adventure?

This list was adapted from a list of family-friendly language for needs that was collected and contributed by Claralynn Nunamaker.

REFERENCES AND RECOMMENDED READING

FOREWORD

References

Page xi: Kitwood, Tom, and Dawn Brooker, eds. *Dementia Reconsidered, Revisited: The Person Still Comes First.* London: Open University Press, 2019.

Page xii: Feil, Naomi. *The Validation Breakthrough: Simple Techniques for Communicating With People With "Alzheimer's-Type Dementia."* Baltimore: Health Professions Press, 1993.

INTRODUCTION: GROWING CONNECTION

References

Page 2:   World Health Organization. "Mental Health." Accessed March 21, 2019. https://www.who.int/mental_health/neurology/dementia/en/

Page 3:   Rogers, Carl. "The Characteristics of a Helping Relationship 1958." In *The Carl Rogers Reader,* edited by Howard Kirschenbaum and Valerie Land Henderson, 108–126. London: Robinson, 1990, page 108.

Page 4:   Center for Nonviolent Communication. "What Is Nonviolent Communication?" Accessed March 21, 2019. https://www.cnvc.org/learn-nvc/what-is-nvc

Page 7:   Philpotts, Eden. *A Shadow Passes.* London: Cecil Palmer & Hayward, 1918, page 19.

CHAPTER 1: ACKNOWLEDGING WHAT'S THERE

References

Page 13:   Le, Xuan, Ian Lancashire, Graeme Hirst, and Regina Jokel. "Longitudinal Detection of Dementia Through Lexical and Syntactic Changes in Writing: A Case Study of Three British Novelists." *Literary*

and Linguistic Computing, Volume 26, Issue 4 (December 2011), pages 435–61. https://doi.org/10.1093/llc/fqr013. See also Day, Adrienne. "Alzheimer's Early Tell: The Language of Authors Who Suffered from Dementia Has a Story for the Rest of Us." *Nautilus*, September 29, 2016. http://nautil.us/issue/40/learning/alzheimers-early-tell.

Page 13: Wikiquote. "Augustine of Hippo." Accessed March 21, 2019. https://en.wikiquote.org/wiki/Augustine_of_Hippo

Page 22: de Mello, Anthony. *The Heart of the Enlightened: A Book of Story Meditations.* New York: Doubleday, 1989, page 146.

Recommended reading

Kitwood, Tom. *Dementia Reconsidered: The Person Comes First.* Buckingham (UK): Open University Press, 1997.

CHAPTER 2: FOCUSING IMAGINATION

References

I have titled each client story in this chapter, in play and with gratitude, after the title of Oliver Sacks's famous book *The Man Who Mistook His Wife for a Hat* (see second note for page 35).

Page 35: Modell, Arnold H. *Imagination and the Meaningful Brain.* Cambridge, MA: MIT Press, 2003, quote by Gerald Edelman on page 37.

Page 35: Sacks, Oliver. *The Man Who Mistook His Wife for a Hat and Other Clinical Tales.* London: Picador, 2011.

Page 43: Ahern, Cecilia. *Love, Rosie.* New York: Hachette, 2005.

Recommended reading

Connor, Jane Marantz, and Dian Killian. *Connecting Across Differences: Finding Common Ground With Anyone, Anywhere, Anytime.* Encinitas, CA: PuddleDancer Press, 2012.

CHAPTER 3: GETTING PERSPECTIVE

References

Page 48: Kitwood, Tom, and Kathleen Bredin. "Tom Kitwood and Kathleen Bredin: 'Towards a Theory of Dementia Care: Personhood and Well-being' (1992). Ageing and Society, 12(3): 269–287." In *Tom Kitwood on Dementia: A Reader and Critical Commentary*, edited by Clive Baldwin and Andrea Capstick, 131–45. London: Open University Press, page 133.

Page 50: Goodreads. "Rumi." Accessed March 21, 2019. https://www.goodreads.com/quotes/245285-you-think-because-you-understand-one-you-must-also-understand

Page 52: PuddleDancer Press. "Marshall Rosenberg's NVC Quotes." Accessed March 21, 2019. https://www.nonviolentcommunication.com/ freeresources/nvc_social_media_quotes.htm

Page 57: Sacks, Oliver. *The Man Who Mistook His Wife for a Hat and Other Clinical Tales*. London: Picador, 2011, page 3.

Page 57: Alzheimer's Association. "Caregivers." Accessed March 21, 2019. https://www.alz.org/professionals/public-health/issues/caregivers

Page 58: Peterson, Christopher, and Martin Seligman. *Character Strengths and Virtues: A Handbook and Classification*. Oxford: Oxford University Press, page 4.

Page 65: Chödrön, Pema. *Comfortable With Uncertainty: 108 Teachings on Cultivating Fearlessness and Compassion*. Boston, MA: Shambhala, 2008, page 74.

Recommended reading

Gonzales, Robert. *Reflections on Living Compassion: Awakening Our Passion and Living in Compassion*. Logan: Utah Publisher's Place, 2015. http://www.living-compassion.org/reflections.html

CHAPTER 4: COMMITTING TO LIFE

References

Page 74: Peyton, Sarah. *Your Resonant Self: Guided Meditations and Exercises to Engage Your Brain's Capacity for Healing*. New York: W. W. Norton & Company, 2017, page 68.

Page 75: Kitwood, Tom, and Kathleen Bredin. "Tom Kitwood and Kathleen Bredin: 'Towards a Theory of Dementia Care: Personhood and Well-being' (1992). Ageing and Society, 12(3): 269–87." In *Tom Kitwood on Dementia: A Reader and Critical Commentary*, edited by Clive Baldwin and Andrea Capstick, 131–45. London: Open University Press, page 133.

Page 77: Elvish, Ruth, Rosanne Cawley, and John Keady. "The Experiences of Counselling and Psychotherapy From the Perspective of Carers of People With Dementia: An Exploration of Client Views and Processes of Change." Lutterworth (UK): British Association for Counselling & Psychotherapy, 2010. Available from: https://www.bacp.co.uk/ media/1976/bacp-experiences-counselling-psychotherapy-from-carers-of-people-with-dementia.pdf

Page 77: Rosenberg, Marshall B. *Nonviolent Communication. A Language of Life*. 3rd edition. Encinitas, CA: PuddleDancer Press, 2015, page 55.

Recommended reading

d'Ansembourg, Thomas. *Being Genuine: Stop Being Nice, Start Being Real.*
        Encinitas, CA: PuddleDancer Press, 2007.

CHAPTER 5: CULTIVATING EMPATHY

References

Page 90:   Peyton, Sarah. *Your Resonant Self: Guided Meditations and Exercises to
        Engage Your Brain's Capacity for Healing.* New York: W. W. Norton &
        Company, 2017, page 62.

Page 94:   This quote is often attributed to Oscar Wilde, which is how I originally
        heard it. However, it turns out there's no good evidence for who said
        it first (see Garson O'Toole, "Be Yourself. Everyone Else Is Already
        Taken," Quote Investigator [website], accessed March 21, 2019,
        https://quoteinvestigator.com/2014/01/20/be-yourself/). Whoever it
        was, I find it a useful message still.

Page 95:   Goodreads. "Steven Wright." Accessed March 21, 2019.
        https://www. goodreads.com/author/quotes/181771.Steven_Wright

Page 100: Peyton, Sarah. *Your Resonant Self: Guided Meditations and Exercises to
        Engage Your Brain's Capacity for Healing.* New York: W. W. Norton &
        Company, 2017.

Recommended reading

Klein, Shari, and Neill Gibson. *What's Making You Angry? 10 Steps to
        Transforming Anger So Everyone Wins.* Encinitas, CA: PuddleDancer
        Press, 2004.

CHAPTER 6: FEEDING INNER POWER

Recommended reading

Rosenberg, Marshall B. *Being Me, Loving You: A Practical Guide to Extraordinary
        Relationships.* Encinitas, CA: PuddleDancer Press, 2005.

CHAPTER 7: SAVORING HURT, GUILT, AND GRIEF

References

Page 121: Larsson, Liv. *The Power of Gratitude.* Svensbyn (Sweden): Friare Liv,
        2014, page 21.

Page 122: Ehrenreich, Barbara. *Bright-Sided: How Positive Thinking Is
        Undermining America.* New York: Metropolitan Books, 2009, page 6.

Page 123: Siegel, Dan. *Mind: A Journey to the Heart of Being Human.* New York:
        W. W. Norton & Company, 2017, page 94.

Page 123: Rosenberg, Marshall B. *Making Life Wonderful: An Intermediate Training in Nonviolent Communication* [DVD]. Albuquerque, NM: Center for Nonviolent Communication . (As of March 21, 2019, this training was viewable on Youtube at https://www.youtube.com/watch?v=LnAEF_TU1z4.)

Page 129: James, William. *Essays and Lectures*, edited by Daniel Kolak. New York: Routledge, 2007, page 143.

Page 131: Mackenzie, Ian, personal communication with the author, March 13, 2019. (My friend Ian is also the author of the chapter "Mindfulness and Presence in Supervision," in *Full Spectrum Supervision: "Who You Are, Is How You Supervise,"* edited by Edna Murdoch, Jackie Arnold, St. Albans (UK): Panoma Press, 2013, pages 121–213.)

Page 134: Hookham, Lama Shenpen. *There Is More to Dying Than Death: A Buddhist Perspective*. Birmingham (UK): Windhorse Publications, 2006, page 174.

Recommended reading

Rosenberg, Marshall B. *Getting Past the Pain Between Us: Healing and Reconciliation Without Compromise*. Encinitas, CA: PuddleDancer Press, 2004.

CHAPTER 8: BEING CURIOUS

References

Page 142: Rosenberg, Marshall B. *Nonviolent Communication: A Language of Life*. 3rd edition. Encinitas, CA: PuddleDancer Press, 2015, quote by Chuang-Tzu on page 91.

Page 145: Koenig Coste, Joanne. *Learning to Speak Alzheimer's: A Groundbreaking Approach for Everyone Dealing With the Disease*. New York: Mariner Books, 2004, page 108.

Page 146: Goodreads. "Ludwig van Beethoven." Accessed March 21, 2019. https://www.goodreads.com/quotes/4103660-to-play-a-wrong-note-is-insignificant-to-play-without

Page 147: Amador, Xavier. *I Am Not Sick, I Don't Need Help!* New York: Vida Press, 2012, page 112.

Page 147: Le, Xuan, Ian Lancashire, Graeme Hirst, and Regina Jokel. "Longitudinal Detection of Dementia Through Lexical and Syntactic Changes in Writing: A Case Study of Three British Novelists." *Literary and Linguistic Computing*, Volume 26, Issue 4 (December 2011), pages 435–61. https://doi.org/10.1093/llc/fqr013. See also Day, Adrienne. "Alzheimer's Early Tell: The Language of Authors Who Suffered from Dementia Has a Story for the Rest of Us." *Nautilus*, September 29, 2016. http://nautil.us/issue/40/learning/alzheimers-early-tell

Page 154: Rogers, Carl. "The Necessary and Sufficient Conditions of Therapeutic Personality Change 1957." In *The Carl Rogers Reader*, edited by Howard Kirschenbaum and Valerie Land Henderson, 219–35. London: Robinson, 1990, page 231.

Page 155: Lipińska, Danuta. *Person-Centred Counselling for People With Dementia: Making Sense of Self.* London: Jessica Kingsley Publishers, 2009, page 9.

Recommended reading

Sears, Melanie. *Choose Your Words: Harnessing the Power of Compassionate Communication to Heal and Connect.* Self-published, CreateSpace, 2015.

CHAPTER 9: TUNING IN TO ANGER AND CONFUSION

Recommended reading

Rosenberg, Marshall B. *The Surprising Purpose of Anger: Beyond Anger Management: Finding the Gift.* Encinitas, CA: PuddleDancer Press, 2005.

CHAPTER 10: ASKING QUESTIONS

References

Page 175: Roth, Philip. *American Pastoral.* London: Vintage Books, 1998, page 55.

Page 181: Mackenzie, Ian, personal communication with the author, March 13, 2019. (My friend Ian is also the author of the chapter "Mindfulness and Presence in Supervision," in *Full Spectrum Supervision: "Who You Are, Is How You Supervise,"* edited by Edna Murdoch, Jackie Arnold, St. Albans (UK): Panoma Press, 2013, pages 121–213.)

Page 181: Jami, Criss. *Healology.* Self-published, 2016, page 6.

Recommended reading

Alzheimer's Society. "Communicating With Someone With Memory Loss." Accessed March 21, 2019. https://www.alzheimers.org.uk/about-dementia/symptoms-and-diagnosis/symptoms/communication-memory-loss

CHAPTER 11: STAYING IN TOUCH

References

Page 185: *Oxford Paperback Dictionary.* Oxford: Oxford University Press, 2009, page 173.

Page 185: Goodreads. "Rumi." Accessed March 21, 2019. https://www.goodreads.com/quotes/117479-words-are-a-pretext-it-is-the-inner-bond-that

Page 188: Goodreads. "Victor Hugo." Accessed March 21, 2019.
https://www.goodreads.com/quotes/14451-music-expresses-that-
which-cannot-be-put-into-words-and

Page 188: Sacks, Oliver. *The Man Who Mistook His Wife for a Hat and Other
Clinical Tales.* London: Picador, 2011.

Page 190: Maitland, Arnaud. *Living Without Regret: Growing Old in the Light of
Tibetan Buddhism.* Casadero, CA: Dharma Publishing, 2005, page 174.

Recommended reading

Mackenzie, Mary. *Peaceful Living: Daily Meditations for Living With Love,
Healing, and Compassion.* Encinitas, CA: PuddleDancer Press, 2005.

ENDNOTE: EXPERIENCING VULNERABILITY

References

Page 194: Lipińska, Danuta. *Person-Centred Counselling for People With
Dementia: Making Sense of Self.* London: Jessica Kingsley Publishers,
2009, page 106.

Page 194: Hookham, Lama Shenpen. *There Is More to Dying Than Death: A
Buddhist Perspective.* Birmingham (UK): Windhorse Publications,
2006.

Page 194: Dass, Ram and Paul Gorman. *How Can I Help? Emotional Support and
Spiritual Inspiration for Those Who Care for Others.* London: Rider,
1986, page 224.

Recommended reading

Hookham, Lama Shenpen. *Living the Awakened Heart.* Self-published,
CreateSpace, 2015.

Rosenberg, Marshall B. *Practical Spirituality: The Spiritual Basis of Nonviolent
Communication.* Encinitas, CA: PuddleDancer Press, 2005.

EPILOGUE: EXPRESSING GRATITUDE WITHOUT A TAIL

References

Page 199: Goodreads. "W.H. Auden." Accessed March 21, 2019.
https://www.goodreads.com/quotes/100377-in-times-of-joy-all-of-us-
wished-we-possessed

Recommended reading

Larsson, Liv. *The Power of Gratitude.* Svensbyn (Sweden): Friare Liv, 2014.

INDEX

A

accusations, 53–59, 158
acknowledgment, need for, 67
aggression, 41–42
Ahern, Cecelia, 43
Amador, Xavier, 147
American Pastoral (Roth), 174–75
anger
    attention and, 157
    grief and, 132
    judgments and, 95
    understanding, 158–64
appreciation, 199
assumptions, 38
attention
    emotions and, 157
    feelings and, 96
    focused, 31
Auden, W.H., 199
Augustine (Saint), 13
avoidance, 128

B

Beattie, Melody, 197
Beethoven, Ludwig van, 146
bereavement, 129–35
Bielak-Smith, Pati, xiv
blame, 53–59, 158
boundaries, 36
Bray-Narai, Paulette, 147
breakdowns, 90
Bredin, Kathleen, 47–48

*Bright-Sided: How the Relentless
    Promotion of Positive Thinking
    Has Undermined America*
    (Ehrenreich), 122

C

caregivers and caregiving
    invisibility of, 18–21
    reasons for, 112
    use of term, 2
    violence toward, 41–42
    well-being of, 57–58, 68
    women as, 77
Center for Nonviolent Communication, 4
Chödrön, Pema, 65, 87
Christie, Agatha, 13
communication. *See* Nonviolent
    Communication
compassion, 65
confusion, 164–69
connections, xv, 23–25, 93, 137, 185.
    See also disconnections
contributions, ability for, 22
Coste, Joanne Koenig, 145

D

Dass, Ram, 194
de Mello, Anthony, 22, 185
death, 193–94
delusions, 23
dementia
    defined, 11–12
    effects of, 23
    statistics on, 2

Dementia Reconsidered (Kitwood), 75
dementia relationships, 6, 47–52, 78–79
depression, 95
diagnosis
    convenience of, 55
    effect of, 14
dis-comfort, 94
dis-connected (disconnected), 23–25,
    71, 90.
    See also connections
disease (dis-ease), xi, xii, 1, 11, 12, 13,
    19, 29, 57, 58, 68, 69, 76, 90,
    154, 184
dis-heartend (disheartened), 71
dis-pleased (displeased), 71
dis-quieted (disquieted), 71
distrust, 54–55
driving ability, 37–38

E
Edelman, Gerald, 35, 171
Ehrenreich, Barbara, 122
emotions
    acknowledgment of, 76
    attention and, 157
    self-empathy and, 90, 95–96.
    See also anger
empathic imagination, 141–43
empathy
    asking for, 101–8
    examples of, 148
    need for, 99–100
    self-empathy, 88–97, 129, 134–35.
    See also self-empathy
English, Elizabeth, 89, 146, 201
equal treatment, 30

F
feeling nothing, 74
feelings
    acknowledgment of, 76
    attention and, 157
    self-empathy and, 90, 95–96.
    See also anger
Feil, Naomi, xiv
flexibility, 36
focused attention, 31

friendships, 33
fulfillment, 74–75

G
giraffe symbol, 46
Gorham, Paul, 194
gratitude, 198–99
grief, 129–35
guessing strategy, 145–51
guilt, 127–29

H
hallucinations, 23
Healology (Jami), 181
heartache, 93–94, 132
hi-story, 173
honesty, 122
Hookham, Lama Shenpen, 134, 194, 201
hope-ful (hopeful), 70
*How Can I Help? Emotional Support and
    Spiritual Inspiration for Those
    Who Care for Others* (Dass
    and Gorham), 194
Hugo, Victor, 188
human needs and values, 60–61
humanistic approach, 3, 154

I
I Am Not Sick, I Don't Need Help!
    (Amador), 147
ill-being, 52, 58, 75
ill-ness (illness), 1–2, 3, 6, 12, 24, 29, 45,
    47, 48, 51, 52, 56, 57, 58, 76,
    98, 123, 134, 137, 142, 147, 154,
    160, 162, 183, 198
imagination
    empathic, 141–43
    need for, 28–30
    trainers in, 30–44
imperfection, 98–101
inclusivity, 122
inner space, 91
inter-presence, 186–87
invisibility
    of caregivers, 18–21
    of those with dementia, 14
Irena (Granny), 15, 20, 193, 195

J

James, William, 129
Jami, Criss, 181
joy-ful (joyful), 70
judgments, 53–59, 94–95, 99

K

Kamieńska, Anna, 121
Kitwood, Tom, xiii, xiv, 47–48, 50, 75, 202
Kristensen, Kirsten, 80

L

language deterioration, 13
language of life, 69–76
Larsson, Liv, 121
Learning to Speak Alzheimer's (Coste), 145
Lem, Stanislaw, 11
Levine, Stephen, 69
Lipińska, Danuta, 155, 194
Living Without Regret (Maitland), 190

M

Macferran, Kathleen, 133–34, 182–83
Mackenzie, Ian, 131, 181
Maitland, Arnaud, 190
The Man Who Mistook His Wife for a Hat (Sacks), 35
Maria (Grandma), 4, 14–17, 20, 22, 131, 177, 193
me-aningful, 173
mechanics analogy, 109–10
memories, 172–77
memory loss, 133
me-story, 173, 175, 176–77,
mistrust, 54–55
moon analogy, 59–60
Murdoch, Iris, 13
music, 187–88

N

needs
    meeting, 70, 74–84, 114–17
    power in, 110–14
    recognition of, 117–20
    universal human, 60–62
    of women, 77
negative thinking, 121–22

neurological function, 57
neutral observations, 140–41
Nietzsche, Friedrich, 139
no, saying, 39–40
Nonviolent Communication
    anger, 160, 162
    communication definition, 185
    discipline of, 21–22
    gratitude, 199
    language of life, 69–76
    perspective and, 46
    practice of, xiv–xv, 5, 46, 119
    process of, 113
    universal human needs, 60–62.
    See also Rosenberg, Marshall B.
nurturing, 109

O

observation of reality, 140–41
overload, 68

P

pain of life, 129
paranormal, 167
passion, 146
peace-ful (peaceful), 33, 70, 71, 114
perceptions, 139–42
person-centered care, xiii
Person-Centered Counseling for People With Dementia: Making Sense of Self (Lipińska), 155
perspective
    dementia relationships and, 78–79
    Nonviolent Communication and, 46
Peterson, Christopher, 58
Peyton, Sarah, 74, 90, 100
physical contact, 188–91
pity, 65
The Places That Scare You: A Guide to Fearlessness in Difficult Times (Chödrön), 65
poignancy, 132–33
positive thinking, 121–22
Pratchett, Terry, 13
presence, 186–87
prevalence of dementia, 2
problems, ownership of, 47–52
Proulx, Annie, 157

Q
questioning, 171–72

R
reality, 117, 140–41, 164–69
recognition, need for, 67
relationship-centered care, xiii
relationships
    dementia relationships, 6, 47–52,
        78–79
    vs. friendships, 33
    Rosenberg, Marshall, on, 52, 123
reorienting to reality, 165, 168–69
repetition, 177–84
requests, refusing, 39
restraints, 161–62
Rogers, Carl, 3, 154
Rosenberg, Marshall B., 109, 193
    giraffe symbol, 46
    on the principles of Nonviolent
        Communication, 4, 62–63
    on relationships, 52, 123
    on women's needs, 77
    See also Nonviolent Communication
Roth, Philip, 174–75
Rumi, 50, 185

S
Sacks, Oliver, 35, 57
sacrifice, 77
sadness
    value of, 131.
    See also grief
scarcity perspective, 57–58
Sears, Melanie, 152, 168–69
sedation, 161–62
self-criticism, 56,
self-empathy, 88–97, 129, 134–35.
    See also empathy
self-judgment, 55.
    See also judgments
Seligman, Martin, 58

Siegel, Daniel J., 123
singing, 188
statistics on dementia, 2
Stead, Rebecca, 45
strategies for meeting needs, 81, 83,
        114–17
suffering, 66
surprises, 107, 145
suspicion, 54–55
symptoms, inconsistency of, 29–30, 51

T
thank-ful (thankful), 70, 71
time, 13
touch, 188–91
trust, 54–55, 188–89
Twain, Mark, 27

U
understanding. See empathy
universal human needs, 60–62

V
values, 60–61
victimhood, 64
violence, 41–42, 161–62
visits from family, 63–64
vocabulary, 13
vulnerability, 94, 123, 132, 193–94

W
wandering, 144
willpower, 97
withdrawal, 75
witnessing, 152–55
women's needs, 77
Woods, Bob, xi–xv
words, loss of, 13
Wright, Steven, 95

Y
Your Resonant Self (Peyton), 74, 90

The Four-Part Nonviolent Communication Process

Clearly expressing how **I am** without blaming or criticizing	Empathically receiving how **you are** without hearing blame or criticism

OBSERVATIONS

1. What I observe *(see, hear, remember, imagine, free from my evaluations)* that does or does not contribute to my well-being:

   "When I (see, hear) . . . "

1. What you observe *(see, hear, remember, imagine, free from your evaluations)* that does or does not contribute to your well-being:

   "When you see/hear . . . "

   (Sometimes unspoken when offering empathy)

FEELINGS

2. How I feel *(emotion or sensation rather than thought)* in relation to what I observe:

   "I feel . . . "

2. How you feel *(emotion or sensation rather than thought)* in relation to what you observe:

   "You feel . . ."

NEEDS

3. What I need or value *(rather than a preference, or a specific action)* that causes my feelings:

   " . . . because I need/value . . . "

3. What you need or value *(rather than a preference, or a specific action)* that causes your feelings:

   " . . . because you need/value . . ."

Clearly requesting that which would enrich **my** life without demanding	Empathically receiving that which would enrich **your** life without hearing any demand

REQUESTS

4. The concrete actions I would like taken:

   "Would you be willing to . . . ?"

4. The concrete actions you would like taken:

   "Would you like . . . ?"

   (Sometimes unspoken when offering empathy)

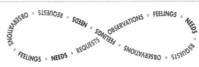

© Marshall B. Rosenberg. For more information about Marshall B. Rosenberg or the Center for Nonviolent Communication, please visit www.CNVC.org.

About Nonviolent Communication

Nonviolent Communication has flourished for more than four decades across sixty countries selling more than 3,000,000 books in over thirty-five languages for one simple reason: it works.

From the bedroom to the boardroom, from the classroom to the war zone, Nonviolent Communication (NVC) is changing lives every day. NVC provides an easy-to-grasp, effective method to get to the root of violence and pain peacefully. By examining the unmet needs behind what we do and say, NVC helps reduce hostility, heal pain, and strengthen professional and personal relationships. NVC is now being taught in corporations, classrooms, prisons, and mediation centers worldwide. And it is affecting cultural shifts as institutions, corporations, and governments integrate NVC consciousness into their organizational structures and their approach to leadership.

Most of us are hungry for skills that can improve the quality of our relationships, to deepen our sense of personal empowerment or simply help us communicate more effectively. Unfortunately, most of us have been educated from birth to compete, judge, demand, and diagnose; to think and communicate in terms of what is "right" and "wrong" with people. At best, the habitual ways we think and speak hinder communication and create misunderstanding or frustration. And still worse, they can cause anger and pain, and may lead to violence. Without wanting to, even people with the best of intentions generate needless conflict.

NVC helps us reach beneath the surface and discover what is alive and vital within us, and how all of our actions are based on human needs that we are seeking to meet. We learn to develop a vocabulary of feelings and needs that helps us more clearly express what is going on in us at any given moment. When we understand and acknowledge our needs, we develop a shared foundation for much more satisfying relationships. Join the thousands of people worldwide who have improved their relationships and their lives with this simple yet revolutionary process.

About PuddleDancer Press

Visit the PDP website at www.NonviolentCommunication.com. We have a resource-rich and ever-growing website that currently addresses 35+ topics related to NVC through articles, online resources, handouts, Marshall Rosenberg quotes, and so much more. Please come visit us.

- **NVC Quick Connect e-Newsletter**—Sign up online to receive our monthly e-Newsletter, filled with expert articles on timely and relevant topics, links to NVC in the news, inspirational and fun quotes and songs, announcements of trainings and other NVC events, and exclusive specials on NVC learning materials.

- **Shop NVC**—Purchase our NVC titles safely, affordably, and conveniently online. Find everyday discounts on individual titles, multiple copies, and book packages. Learn more about our authors and read endorsements of NVC from world-renowned communication experts and peacemakers.

- **About NVC**—Learn more about the unique life-changing communication and conflict resolution skills of NVC (also known as Compassionate Communication, Collaborative Communication, Respectful Communication, Mindful Communication, Peaceful Communication, or Effective Communication). Find an overview of the NVC process, key facts about NVC, and more.

- **About Marshall Rosenberg**—Read about the world-renowned peacemaker, educator, best-selling author, and founder of the Center for Nonviolent Communication, including press materials, a biography, and more.

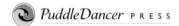

For more information, please contact PuddleDancer Press at:

2240 Encinitas Blvd., Ste. D-911 • Encinitas, CA 92024
Phone: 760-652-5754 • Fax: 760-274-6400
Email: email@puddledancer.com • www.NonviolentCommunication.com

223

About the Center for Nonviolent Communication

The Center for Nonviolent Communication (CNVC) is an international nonprofit peacemaking organization whose vision is a world where everyone's needs are met peacefully. CNVC is devoted to supporting the spread of Nonviolent Communication (NVC) around the world.

Founded in 1984 by Dr. Marshall B. Rosenberg, CNVC has been contributing to a vast social transformation in thinking, speaking and acting—showing people how to connect in ways that inspire compassionate results. NVC is now being taught around the globe in communities, schools, prisons, mediation centers, churches, businesses, professional conferences, and more. Hundreds of certified trainers and hundreds more supporters teach NVC to tens of thousands of people each year in more than sixty countries.

CNVC believes that NVC training is a crucial step to continue building a compassionate, peaceful society. Your tax-deductible donation will help CNVC continue to provide training in some of the most impoverished, violent corners of the world. It will also support the development and continuation of organized projects aimed at bringing NVC training to high-need geographic regions and populations.

To make a tax-deductible donation or to learn more about the valuable resources described below, visit the CNVC website at www. CNVC.org:

- **Training and Certification**—Find local, national, and international training opportunities, access trainer certification information, connect to local NVC communities, trainers, and more.

- **CNVC Bookstore**—Find mail or phone order information for a complete selection of NVC books, booklets, audio, and video materials at the CNVC website.

- **CNVC Projects**—Participate in one of the several regional and theme-based projects that provide focus and leadership for teaching NVC in a particular application or geographic region.

For more information, please contact CNVC at:

Ph: 505-244-4041 • US Only: 800-255-7696 • Fax: 505-247-0414
Email: cnvc@CNVC.org • Website: www.CNVC.org

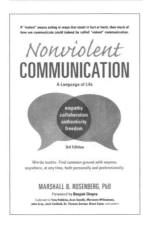

Nonviolent Communication,

3rd Edition

A Language of Life

By Marshall B. Rosenberg, PhD

$19.95 — Trade Paper 6x9, 264pp
ISBN: 978-1-892005-28-1

What is Violent Communication?

If "violent" means acting in ways that result in hurt or harm, then much of how we communicate —judging others, bullying, having racial bias, blaming, finger pointing, discriminating, speaking without listening, criticizing others or ourselves, name-calling, reacting when angry, using political rhetoric, being defensive or judging who's "good/ bad" or what's "right/wrong" with people—**could indeed be called "violent communication."**

What is Nonviolent Communication?

Nonviolent Communication is the integration of four things:

- **Consciousness: a set of principles that support living a life of compassion, collaboration, courage, and authenticity**
- **Language: understanding how words contribute to connection or distance**
- **Communication: knowing how to ask for what we want, how to hear others even in disagreement, and how to move toward solutions that work for all**
- **Means of influence: sharing "power with others" rather than using "power over others"**

Nonviolent Communication serves our desire to do three things:

- **Increase our ability to live with choice, meaning, and connection**
- **Connect empathically with self and others to have more satisfying relationships**
- **Sharing of resources so everyone is able to benefit**

Available from PuddleDancer Press, the Center for Nonviolent Communication, all major bookstores, and Amazon.com. Distributed by Independent Publisher's Group: 800-888-4741. For Best Pricing Visit: NonviolentCommunication.com

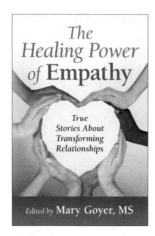

The Healing Power of Empathy

True Stories About Transforming Relationships

Edited by Mary Goyer, MS

$17.95 – Trade Paper 6x9, 288pp
ISBN: 978-1-934336-17-5

Empathy Is a Learnable Skill!

Empathy is the cornerstone of good relationships—but it can be hard to access when it's most needed. Luckily, empathy is also a learnable skill, with the power to move conversations out of gridlock and pain.

- You'll see how anger and blame get translated and how productive dialogues are made possible.
- You'll hear the words used to repair arguments before they cause damage.
- You'll watch how self-empathy transforms relationships—without speaking any words at all.

"Our ability to offer empathy can allow us to stay vulnerable, defuse potential violence, help us hear the word no without taking it as a rejection, revive lifeless conversation, and even hear the feelings and needs expressed through silence. The best way I can get understanding from another person is to give this person the understanding too. If I want them to hear my needs and feelings, I first need to empathize."

—**Marshall B. Rosenberg, PhD**, Author and Creator of Nonviolent Communication, over 3,000,000 copies sold worldwide

"Each vignette provides a living example of the transformative power of this special form of listening and being. Every story, in its own way, gives a hopeful glimpse of a world where people deeply care for one another and express that caring through their language. This book inspires me to bring more empathy into my life and work to make this world a reality."

—**David McCain**, Trainer, Coach, Consultant, and CNVC Certification Candidate

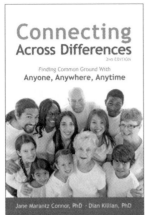

Connecting Across Differences, 2nd Edition

Finding Common Ground With Anyone, Anywhere, Anytime

By Jane Marantz Connor, PhD and Dian Killian, PhD

$19.95 — Trade Paper 6x9, 416pp
ISBN: 978-1-892005-24-3

Profound Connection Is Just a Conversation Away!

In this fully revised second edition, Dr. Dian Killian and Dr. Jane Marantz Connor offer a comprehensive and accessible guide for exploring the concepts, applications, and transformative power of the Nonviolent Communication process. Discover simple, yet transformative skills to create a life of abundance, where building the personal, professional, and community connections you long for begins with a simple shift in thinking.

Now with an expanded selection of broadly applicable exercises, role-plays, and activities that challenge readers to immediately apply the concepts in everyday life, this new edition opens the authors' insight to an even broader audience. Detailed and comprehensive, this combined book and workbook enhances communication skills by introducing the basic NVC model, as well as more advanced NVC practices. Relevant, meaningful exercises follow each concept, giving readers the chance to immediately apply the skills they've learned to real life experiences.

Drawing on a combined 25 years of experience, the authors help readers to:
- Transform negative self-talk into self empowerment
- Foster trust and collaboration when stakes are high
- Establish healthy relationships to satisfy your needs
- Defuse anger, enemy images, and other barriers to connection
- Get what you want while maintaining respect and integrity

In each chapter, numerous exercises invite readers to apply NVC skills and concepts in their own lives. The second part features extensive dialogues illustrating NVC in action including in self-empathy, empathy, and mediation. The book closes with a resource guide for further learning and an interview with Marshall Rosenberg from the February 2003 *Sun Magazine.*

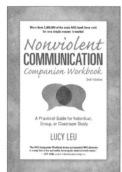

Nonviolent Communication
Companion Workbook, 2nd Edition
A Practical Guide for Individual, Group, or Classroom Study

By Lucy Leu

$21.95 — Trade Paper 7x10, 240pp
ISBN: 978-1-892005-29-8

Putting NVC Skills Into Practice!

Learning Nonviolent Communication has often been equated with learning a whole new language. *The NVC Companion Workbook* helps you put these powerful, effective skills into practice with chapter-by-chapter study of Marshall Rosenberg's cornerstone text, *NVC: A Language of Life*. Create a safe, supportive group learning or practice environment that nurtures the needs of each participant. Find a wealth of activities, exercises, and facilitator suggestions to refine and practice this powerful communication process.

Nonviolent Communication has flourished for more than four decades across sixty countries selling more than 3,000,000 books for a simple reason: it works.

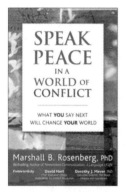

Speak Peace in a World of Conflict
What You Say Next Will Change Your World

By Marshall B. Rosenberg, PhD

$15.95 — Trade Paper 5-3/8x8-3/8, 208pp
ISBN: 978-1-892005-17-5

Create Peace in the Language You Use!

International peacemaker, mediator, and healer, Marshall Rosenberg shows you how the language you use is the key to enriching life. *Speak Peace* is filled with inspiring stories, lessons, and ideas drawn from more than forty years of mediating conflicts and healing relationships in some of the most war-torn, impoverished, and violent corners of the world. Find insight, practical skills, and powerful tools that will profoundly change your relationships and the course of your life for the better.

Nonviolent Communication has flourished for more than four decades across sixty countries selling more than 3,000,000 books for a simple reason: it works.

Available from PuddleDancer Press, the Center for Nonviolent Communication, all major bookstores, and Amazon.com. Distributed by Independent Publisher's Group: 800-888-4741. For Best Pricing Visit: NonviolentCommunication.com

228

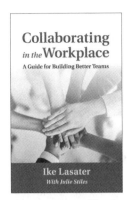

Collaborating in the Workplace
A Guide for Building Better Teams

By Ike Lasater
With Julie Stiles

$7.95 — Trade Paper 5-3/8x8-3/8, 88pp
ISBN: 978-1-934336-16-8

Foster Superior Collaboration!

What can individuals do to improve the ability of teams to collaborate and create powerful outcomes? *Collaborating in the Workplace* focuses on the key skills that research shows support effective collaboration and the practical, step-by-step exercises that individuals can practice to improve those skills. By using this book, people can work better together to create outstanding outcomes.

"A wonderfully practical guide for building teams and getting the best out of everyone. If you are looking to build collaboration in the workplace, start by reading this book!"

—**Daniel L. Shapiro, PhD**, Author of *Negotiating the Nonnegotiable*

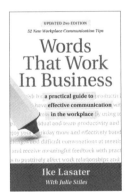

Words That Work In Business,
Updated 2nd Edition
A Practical Guide to Effective Communication in the Workplace

By Ike Lasater
With Julie Stiles

$15.95 — Trade Paper 5-3/8x8-3/8, 208pp
ISBN: 978-1-934336-15-1

Be Happier and More Effective at Work!

Words That Work in Business, 2nd edition, is a must-have guide to thriving in the workplace. Learn how to reduce workplace conflict and stress, effectively handle difficult conversations, have more effective meetings, give and receive meaningful feedback, and navigate power differentials, all of which serve to improve your productivity and fulfillment.

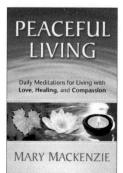

Peaceful Living
Daily Meditations for Living With Love, Healing, and Compassion

By Mary Mackenzie

$19.95 — Trade Paper 5x7.5, 448pp
ISBN: 978-1-892005-19-9

Live More Authentically and Peacefully Than You Ever Dreamed Possible

In this gathering of wisdom, Mary Mackenzie empowers you with an intimate life map that will literally change the course of your life for the better. Each of the 366 meditations includes an inspirational quote and concrete, practical tips for integrating the daily message into your life. The learned behaviors of cynicism, resentment, and getting even are replaced with the skills of Nonviolent Communication, including recognizing one's needs and values and making choices in alignment with them.

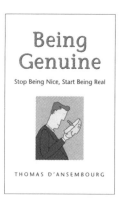

Being Genuine
Stop Being Nice, Start Being Real

By Thomas d'Ansembourg

$17.95 — Trade Paper 5-3/8x8-3/8, 280pp
ISBN: 978-1-892005-21-2

A Fresh, New Perspective on Communication!

Being Genuine brings Thomas d'Ansembourg's blockbuster French title to the English market. His work offers you a fresh new perspective on the proven skills offered in the bestselling book, *Nonviolent Communication: A Language of Life*. Drawing on his own real-life examples and stories, Thomas d'Ansembourg provides practical skills and concrete steps that allow us to safely remove the masks we wear, which prevent the intimacy and satisfaction we desire with our intimate partners, children, parents, friends, family, and colleagues.

"Through this book, we can feel Nonviolent Communication not as a formula but as a rich, meaningful way of life, both intellectually and emotionally."

—**Vicki Robin**, cofounder, Conversation Cafes, coauthor, *Your Money or Your Life*

Based on Marshall Rosenberg's Nonviolent Communication process

Available from PuddleDancer Press, the Center for Nonviolent Communication, all major bookstores, and Amazon.com. Distributed by Independent Publisher's Group: 800-888-4741. For Best Pricing Visit: NonviolentCommunication.com

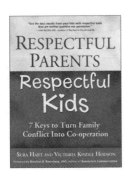

Respectful Parents, Respectful Kids
7 Keys to Turn Family Conflict Into Co-operation

By Sura Hart and Victoria Kindle Hodson

$17.95 — Trade Paper 7.5x9.25, 256pp
ISBN: 978-1-892005-22-9

Stop the Struggle—Find the Co-operation and Mutual Respect You Want!

Do more than simply correct bad behavior—finally unlock your parenting potential. Use this handbook to move beyond typical discipline techniques and begin creating an environment based on mutual respect, emotional safety, and positive, open communication. *Respectful Parents, Respectful Kids* offers *7 Simple Keys* to discover the mutual respect and nurturing relationships you've been looking for.

Use these 7 Keys to:
- Set firm limits without using demands or coercion
- Achieve mutual respect without being submissive
- Successfully prevent, reduce, and resolve conflicts
- Make your home a *No-Fault Zone* where trust thrives

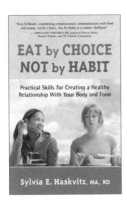

Eat by Choice, Not by Habit
Practical Skills for Creating a Healthy Relationship With Your Body and Food

By Sylvia Haskvitz, MA, RD

$8.95 — 5-3/8x8-3/8, 128pp
ISBN: 978-1-892005-20-5

Develop a Healthy Relationship With Food!

Eating is a basic human need. But what if you are caught up in the cycles of overconsumption or emotional eating? Using the consciousness of Nonviolent Communication, *Eat by Choice* helps you dig deeper into the emotional consciousness that underlies your eating patterns. Much more than a prescriptive fad diet, you'll learn practical strategies to develop a healthier relationship with food. Learn to enjoy the tastes, smells, and sensations of healthful eating once again.

"Face Your Stuff, or Stuff Your Face"

—anonymous

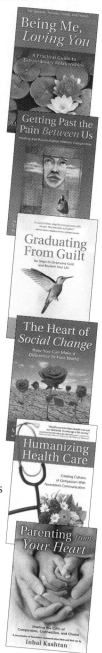

Being Me, Loving You: *A Practical Guide to Extraordinary Relationships* **by Marshall B. Rosenberg, PhD** • Watch your relationships strengthen as you learn to think of love as something you "do," something you give freely from the heart.
80pp, ISBN: 978-1-892005-16-8 • **$6.95**

Getting Past the Pain Between Us: *Healing and Reconciliation Without Compromise* **by Marshall B. Rosenberg, PhD** • Learn simple steps to create the heartfelt presence necessary for lasting healing to occur—great for mediators, counselors, families, and couples.
48pp, ISBN: 978-1-892005-07-6 • **$6.95**

Graduating From Guilt: *Six Steps to Overcome Guilt and Reclaim Your Life* **by Holly Michelle Eckert** • The burden of guilt leaves us stuck, stressed, and feeling like we can never measure up. Through a proven six-step process, this book helps liberate you from the toxic guilt, blame, and shame you carry.
96pp, ISBN: 978-1-892005-23-6 • **$7.95**

The Heart of Social Change: *How to Make a Difference in Your World* **by Marshall B. Rosenberg, PhD** • Learn how creating an internal consciousness of compassion can impact your social change efforts.
48pp, ISBN: 978-1-892005-10-6 • **$6.95**

Humanizing Health Care: *Creating Cultures of Compassion With Nonviolent Communication* **by Melanie Sears, RN, MBA, PhD** • Leveraging more than twenty-five years nursing experience, Melanie demonstrates the profound effectiveness of NVC to create lasting, positive improvements to patient care and the health care workplace.
112pp, ISBN: 978-1-892005-26-7 • **$7.95**

Parenting From Your Heart: *Sharing the Gifts of Compassion, Connection, and Choice* **by Inbal Kashtan** • Filled with insight and practical skills, this booklet will help you transform your parenting to address every day challenges.
48pp, ISBN: 978-1-892005-08-3 • **$6.95**

Practical Spirituality: *Reflections on the Spiritual Basis of Nonviolent Communication* **by Marshall B. Rosenberg, PhD** • Marshall's views on the spiritual origins and underpinnings of NVC, and how practicing the process helps him connect to the Divine.
48pp, ISBN: 978-1-892005-14-4 • **$6.95**

Raising Children Compassionately: *Parenting the Nonviolent Communication Way* **by Marshall B. Rosenberg, PhD** • Learn to create a mutually respectful, enriching family dynamic filled with heartfelt communication.
32pp, ISBN: 978-1-892005-09-0 • **$5.95**

The Surprising Purpose of Anger: *Beyond Anger Management: Finding the Gift* **by Marshall B. Rosenberg, PhD** • Marshall shows you how to use anger to discover what you need, and then how to meet your needs in more constructive, healthy ways.
48pp, ISBN: 978-1-892005-15-1 • **$6.95**

Teaching Children Compassionately: *How Students and Teachers Can Succeed With Mutual Understanding* **by Marshall B. Rosenberg, PhD** • In this national keynote address to Montessori educators, Marshall describes his progressive, radical approach to teaching that centers on compassionate connection.
48pp, ISBN: 978-1-892005-11-3 • **$6.95**

We Can Work It Out: *Resolving Conflicts Peacefully and Powerfully* **by Marshall B. Rosenberg, PhD** • Practical suggestions for fostering empathic connection, genuine co-operation, and satisfying resolutions in even the most difficult situations.
32pp, ISBN: 978-1-892005-12-0 • **$5.95**

What's Making You Angry? *10 Steps to Transforming Anger So Everyone Wins* **by Shari Klein and Neill Gibson** • A powerful, step-by-step approach to transform anger to find healthy, mutually satisfying outcomes.
32pp, ISBN: 978-1-892005-13-7 • **$5.95**

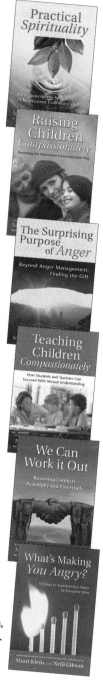

Available from www.NonviolentCommunication.com, www.CNVC.org, Amazon.com and all bookstores. Distributed by IPG: 800-888-4741. For Best Pricing Visit: NonviolentCommunication.com

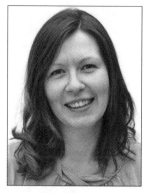

ABOUT THE AUTHOR

Pati Bielak-Smith first witnessed the power of Nonviolent Communication (NVC) to repair and deepen relationships in 2006. Following intensive NVC training in the United Kingdom and in Poland, her motherland, she became a certified trainer with the international Center for Nonviolent Communication in 2014. While studying NVC, she spent five years as a private caregiver for people with dementia who lived alone in their homes.

Caregiving gave Pati the opportunity to see firsthand how the principles of NVC could be used to support everyone living with dementia. Pati has since trained caregivers and supported family members to connect to people living with dementia and, as a Dementia Champion with the Alzheimer's Society, has facilitated dementia information sessions for the community. She has also worked as a meditation teacher and as a communication consultant and trainer for organizations both large and small.

Pati has a master's degree in philosophy and a Diploma in Therapeutic Counselling. She is a member of the British Association for Counselling and Psychotherapy and currently offers one-to-one therapy sessions online or in person through her private practice, which specializes in bringing together NVC and person-centered therapy. Pati lives with her husband in Wales, United Kingdom, where together they devote their personal life to the practice of meditation.

For more information, visit
www.bielaksmith.com/dementiatogether.